PUTAS OF THE CARIBBEAN

(PROSTITUTES OF THE CARIBBEAN)

LEO ALEXANDER

SECOND EDITION

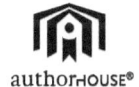

authorHOUSE®

AuthorHouse™
1663 Liberty Drive
Bloomington, IN 47403
www.authorhouse.com
Phone: 1-800-839-8640

Published by AuthorHouse 10/11/2012

ISBN: 978-1-4634-0523-6 (sc)
ISBN: 978-1-4634-0524-3 (e)

Library of Congress Control Number: 2011910013

EDITOR HELEN MILSOM

ABOUT THE AUTHOR

Leo Alexander was born in 1962 in Durban, South Africa. He had a strict Catholic upbringing, and attended church every week of his life up until the age of 17. In 1988 he moved to the Caribbean, where he lived on the island of Curacao before immigrating to Canada in 2007.

ABOUT THE BOOK

In this provocative and enlightening story collection, journey inside the world of legal prostitution. Based on true events, Putas of the Caribbean takes you inside the lives and experiences of prostitutes working in the Caribbean. Read their stories and those of their clients in this intriguing collection. The practice of voluntary prostitution is accepted in many areas around the globe and is completely legal and accepted in many islands of the Caribbean. The following is based on true events that take you into the lives and experiences of prostitutes and their clients in the Caribbean, most of which occurred in Curacao. There are stories from friends, acquaintances, and most of important of all, the girls who actually had sex for money. The events and stories span over a period of about 21 years. Only a few men like Alexander have ever been able to break through the protective barriers the women put up, thus entering hearts, minds and souls of the "working girls". All women featured in this book were over the legal age of 18 and to the best of my knowledge were not forced into prostitution.

Special Thanks

I would like to thank the following people who generously gave me their input and support while writing this book. This book would not have been possible without the women I write about who were willing to allow me some insight to their lives and experiences. To Juan Carlos and others for all their stories. My editor, Helen, who helped make the book appeal to both sexes. Lastly, I will be forever grateful to my late wife for putting up with me for all those years.

TABLE OF CONTENTS

CHAPTER 1
WELCOME TO THE CARIBBEAN

I t was in 1988 and I was 26 when I left the world I knew in South Africa and flew to the Island of Saint Maarten in the Caribbean. A beautiful ground hostess named Lisa checked me in on the Eastern Airlines flight in Miami bound for St. Maarten. She was interested and intrigued with me as I had come from Africa and she hoped to go there one day. We exchanged contact information, but we never saw each other again. I wonder if she ever made it to Africa.

When I arrived in Saint Maarten and stepped off the plane I was immediately greeted by the Island heat and knew, *"hey mun tis da Caribbean"*. Leaving the airport I passed by old colonial style houses as the taxi took me down to the city of Phillipsburg. The Island is half Dutch and half French. Phillipsburg is located on the Dutch side. When St. Maarten was first settled it is said that the French and Dutch decided to share the

Island. So a Frenchman and a Dutchman decided to start at a certain point of the Island, each one walking in opposite directions around the islands' coast. At the point where they met up they drew a line across to split the Island in two. They say the Dutchman stopped along the way for drinks and that is why the Dutch side is smaller than the French. Well, that's the simple version of the story anyway.

There were a lot of sailors, better known as "yachtees" on the Island. Many of them would visit a pub called Sam's Place. It was well known to the crew of cruise ships as well. The original owner, a South African, was killed in a light aircraft accident in the Caribbean. I headed straight over to check it out. Over a few drinks I met a Swedish guy there named Mark, who later became a good friend.

He directed me to a guesthouse on Back Street where I had to pay $20 a night. The room did not have air conditioning, but a big ceiling fan which managed to keep me cool at night. I was also introduced to "Island style" of no hot water in the showers. This was fine though as the temperature would average about 32 degrees Celsius. The water is generally warm or lukewarm as the pipes are close to the surface, enabling the hot Caribbean sun to heat the water.

One day Martin and I decided to rent scooters and take a ride around the Island. We were just leaving Phillipsburg when we noticed a place along the road full of hot women hanging around outside. With free time on our hands, curious and single we decided we just had to stop and investigate. We parked our scooters out front and entered the establishment. Entering the bar we walked over to the bar counter located on the opposite side of the entrance and to the left. On the right was a small stage and dance floor. The place was not too large, just a comfortable size. We ordered ice cold Amstel beers to quench our thirst from the Caribbean heat. I sat down, looked around, and noticed about 12 women in the bar. We soon discovered that they were all Latinos. It was not long when a hot looking young woman came over and introduced herself to me.

She spoke Spanish. At that stage of my life the only Spanish I knew was "si" or "no". She surprised me by beginning to rub my crotch and of course gave me an instant hard on. I had not had any sex in a while because of the traveling. She became excited as she rubbed my cock, which was protruding straight out due to lose thin shorts I was wearing. She called over to her friends saying something in Spanish. I can only guess she said something about my stiff cock. Three girls came over and one by one they each took turns squeezing their hands around my cock. I felt like it was almost as if they were shaking hands with my dick and implying **"Welcome To the Caribbean"**. I sat back and enjoyed this unorthodox greeting.

This turned out to be the Seaman's Club, a well-known whorehouse in Saint Maarten. That day I had my first Latino puta in the Caribbean named Sandra, a 19 year old Colombian. She was a hot looking young woman with long dark hair, rounded curvy body, and nice firm tits. She hadn't had children before so her pussy was nice and tight. She was dressed in her day time sporty attire, tight white shorts, blue stripped top and sneakers. Cost back then was only US $20. A great value for the money.

The first Spanish word a westerner learns is **"Cuanto"** which means "How Much?" Followed by two other words you would hear as a response: "Cincuenta" = Fifty and "Cien" = One hundred. This is generally the going rate for a hookers in the Caribbean.

CHAPTER 2
WORK PLACES

I n many places throughout the Caribbean and Latin America prostitution is legal or tolerated. Work places in these parts consist of bars, whorehouses, nightclubs, taverns, street, casinos and hotel lobbies. Like many places in the world, most islands in the Caribbean will have a place to visit. However you will find that the working girls typically come from other Islands or South America.

In Dominican Republic they have turned some residential homes into high-class whorehouses. The houses look like ordinary homes in the area, and only the taxi drivers or their clients would know where they are. The women plying their trade in these circumstances are mainly beautiful Dominican women. Some of them are women who have boyfriends or are married. Their boyfriends or husbands would drop them off for work in the evening and pick them up in the morning. It was not uncommon to witness a scooter pulling up to the house with the man driving and their woman on the back all dressed up ready for work.

"Casablanca" or "White House" is one of these houses. Situated in a residential area of Santiago, Dominican Republic's second largest city. Home to many beautiful fair skinned Dominican women. I was quite taken with the place from the moment we entered. The host directed us out along a paved pathway to the garden. We were led to a table surrounded by plants, blocking the view of the house. With a clear star lit sky above, this was a lovely tranquil and comfortable setting. After having been served drinks, the host came back out around the corner along the path followed by an entourage of women. One by one he introduced each of the beautiful women to us. We felt like Kings relaxing in the garden atmosphere being presented with female offerings. The place was known for beautiful and quality women. There was even talk of some Canadian women working at Casablanca at times.

Another common place in the Dominican Republic is in the nightclubs. Most of the nightclubs also have shows, from stripteases to cabaret. The problem is that if you take one of the girls you have to pay the house a fee. Normally you would take the woman to a motel, of which there are plenty all over the cities. These motels are very clean, discrete and well organized.

You would drive into the premises, park your car in an open garage, and close the door behind you. Then enter the room through the garage. The telephone would ring and an operator then asks if you require anything to drink. A few minutes later your drinks arrive, usually a bottle of rum, cokes and a bucket of ice. The drinks are passed through a revolving hatch, so that you do not see each other. You then pay for the drinks and the room. Most rooms have a large comfortable bed, Jacuzzi and porno movies showing on the TV. Many motels have a theme or have their own distinctive design. Their brightly lit signs attract the attention of anyone passing by.

I recall a time sitting in the Jacuzzi in one of these places drinking champagne, porno movie showing and two hot Dominican girls having a go at each other on the bed. One was lying on her back legs apart, while the other licked away on her pussy. While sitting back with a drink in hand I couldn't but think to myself, "Man, this is the life". Of course I later joined in on the fun. I ended up eating the one woman's pussy while the other was sucking my cock without a condom. She had beautiful long red fingernails with soft hands that were caressing me. Then she did something that was new to me at that time. She sucked hard on my cock then slid part of her finger up my ass. I could not contain myself and shot a full load of cum into her mouth. The girl on top of me was in ecstasy as I tried to push her away. I wanted to see the reaction of the girl with her mouth full of cum. However she held on to me, pussy pressed tight against my mouth. I was unable to see how the other girl had reacted.

Ah, but I digress. Must get back to places of business. The Carwash is a place you must experience in Dominican Republic. Yes, it is an actual carwash, with an open air bar and patio. Drop your cars off for a wash and spend the time on the patio with plenty of girls for companionship. You can order the drinks by the bottle, generally scotch or rum. Some places you can only take the women away after their shift is finished. Others will have rooms around the back or you can take them to a nearby motel. Most of the time guys just go there for the drinks and company of the women. You'll hear Latina music usually blaring in the background, and an area where you can dance with the girls.

Street hookers are not too common as authorities prefer the women to be working in designated areas. In many places you have to be careful as some street hookers are not women, but transvestites or transsexuals. Some are even prettier than the women. San Juan, Puerto Rico is a place you will find these kinds of "girls" on the street. I passed by some of them on Ponce Leon, a street near the hotel where I was staying. Some of them would flash their tits at me, saying to me in Spanish "look at this Papi". Surprisingly natural looking tits I must say.

One of the famous places in Puerto Rico was the Black Angus, which has since been closed down. The girls would always try the same trick. As soon as you have the girl in the room, her friend would come knocking or storm into the room and ask if you wanted a threesome. This ploy, obviously to gain more money, was also used in some of the guesthouses in Curaçao.

When I was visiting Tegucigalpa in Honduras, I saw some street hookers near the hotel I was staying at and was curious about how much they charged. As I approached them, a pretty brunette eyed me and approached. She suggested I walk with her. I turned around with her by my side and headed towards the direction of the hotel. She was walking as fast as she could as I was questioning her on her services. I then heard calls from behind me as we reached the corner. Five other women were calling out to me in Spanish, "Choose me. I am the one for you". The girl by my side called backed to them and said that I had chosen her. All I was doing was inquiring about the services. I called back that I was not interested, but they kept on pursuing me, saying that they were the girl for me. Eventually I turned to the girl by my side and told her I was not interested and started to run. I looked back and saw all 6 girls running after me. At this point I was worried what the hotel guests and staff would think of me running to the hotel with all these women in pursuit. Luckily, as I approached the hotel, they backed off. Never had I met such desperate hookers. There too I was told by locals that not all the streetwalkers were girls.

Later in my room I got to thinking about what happened. I had a curious thought, what would have happened if I took the brunette back with me? As she took off her panties, would she have exposed a cleanly shaved pussy ready to be penetrated or would she have pulled out a cock? Hmm.

The most famous of all places in the Caribbean is located on the Dutch Island of Curacao. **Campo Alegre**. It is situated on top of the hill overlooking the Hato airport. Campo Alegre's name was changed to Mirage for a while, but returned to the original name of Campo Alegre. Most likely as everyone would still refer to it as Campo. Other names or phrases used are "On the hill" or "The library" It was commonly called these by friends of mine. The name was used as you would be able to speak openly about it without wives or girlfriends really knowing what you are talking about. "Going up the road tonight?", "Read any good books lately?" or "I read a great book at the library the other night."

Campo Alegre is believed to have started after WW11. A friend of mine had an uncle who had visited Campo soon after the war. There are two stories of how or why this place began. One was that it was established by the local authorities because of the large presence of foreign employees who worked at the Shell Oil Refinery. It was thought that horny young single men would not screw their daughters, but instead would visit the whores. The second story is that the first women to work in this place were prisoners at that time. They were given the opportunity to work off their sentences and make some money at the same time. The latter version proved to be false after I met with one of the owners.

The first women ever to work at Campo were from Cuba. One of the Cuban Ministers commented back then that they had the most beautiful putas in the world. This was before the Cuban revolution that occurred in the 1950s. Fidel Castro put a stop to Cuban women working at Campo. Since then Campo has always had the worldwide reputation of having beautiful women, mostly Latinos.

Campo was in fact an old army camp that was turned into a legally run whorehouse with a total of 150 rooms, each with their own bathrooms consisting of a toilet, shower unit and wash basin. In the past, these rooms were not air-conditioned but with fans. The girls had to buy the fans for themselves or were passed on to the next woman.

There was dirt in between the barracks, so you knew if someone had visited Campo just by looking at his shoes. As dust would cover your shoes someone would notice and remark "Hey you just been to

Campo?" There was an old sign at the gate that read "For men only. No women or dogs allowed"

The place went through major renovations starting in the late 1990's. With all the rooms fitted with air-conditioners and TV's showing porno movies. Palm trees were planted along with other tropical plants. All the areas between the rooms have now been paved. Each room is also fitted with a panic button. If a woman feels she is in any danger she can press it and within minutes a security guard will be at her door. On the outside, a red light is fitted above each door. The switch is located on the inside of the doorway, so when switched on it is to indicate the woman is occupied. Some rooms are like a small one bedroom apartment. The front room typically consists of only a chair or small sofa. Some women place their CD players in this room. Then going through a doorway into a small bedroom about 8' x 8' with the bathroom on the side. Some have glass shower units in the bedroom, so the client can watch the woman shower. All bedrooms are fitted with a large mirror on the wall next to the bed.

A large bar with pool tables and slot machines is located in the middle of the grounds. They qualified for a Casino license as they met the minimum number of 100 rooms a hotel is required to have a license. Later the Casino was closed down due to a new licensing regulation.

The Casino primarily had the German Bergmann roulettes. We would bet 3 Guilders on a number and if your number came up, you would win back 36 guilders. This was just enough to pay for a quickie. The joke was that every visit we would try our luck to see if we get a 3 guilder fuck.

In the future, they plan to build a swimming pool for the girls and customers. There was a lot of controversy about all these renovations, which ran into the millions of guilders. One of the owners and his lawyer served out a prison term for organized crime and money laundering. The former Minister of Justice was implicated for giving special work permits for the girls. He soon died after his arrest, which is still under investigation as to the cause of death. I speculate it was stress brought on by his arrest.

There was a period of time when the girls were unable to get work permits. The Lieutenant Governor refused to give the girls' work permits because of illegal permits the former Justice Minister had issued. The authorities wanted to ship all the girls back to their own countries as they had declared their permits were illegal. All the hookers filed suit against the Government and won the case to continue working. They claimed they did not know their permits were illegal. Campo owners also said that if the girls were not able to get work permits, they would start hiring local girls to do the work. Surprisingly they did get some local applications. We'll discuss this point more later on. The Lawyer who had represented the girls and won the case for them was treated to a private show. He was a little embarrassed as he did not expect this. As he sat in a chair they danced all around him, stripping off their clothes.

Soon all was resolved and the court case against Campo resulted with a hefty fine and reduced prison terms. The place returned back to normal, with plenty of girls of your choice to suit your taste. Short, tall, fat, thin, light, dark . . . . all shapes and sizes. There have been look-a-likes, like Shakira and even Monica Lewinski. The Monica look-a-like had no clue who Monica Lewinski was when we told her who she looked like. She probably wondered why so many men had requested a blowjob and wanted to cum on her dress.

In February 2009 the owner of Campo was gunned down outside a supermarket at about 6.05pm. His grandfather was one of the founding partners of Campo. He had recently been released from jail after serving many years for money laundering. The case was still under investigation. Some claim it was to do with the ongoing lawsuit on the ownership of campo as his lawyer had taken over running of the place while he was in jail. There were also rumors about Dutch Mafia involved. Another theory was that it could have been a revenge attack from one of the family members that he had arranged to be eliminated in the past.

He had a long lease on the property, the land and buildings actually belonged to the Government.

The new owners were able to take over ownership by purchasing the land and buildings from the Government. It is believed that the property was valued at 6.5 million Guilders (3.6 million US Dollars). They had made an offer of 250,000 guilders but was eventually settled for 2.5 million Guilders.

Most of the girls working at Campo come from Dominican Republic, Colombia and occasionally from Brazil, Ecuador or Costa Rica. Recently my friends and I came across a Russian woman who was brought in to teach the women to dance for the nightly shows. Nowadays you will find mostly Colombian women work at Campo. They come for a three month contract. In order to gain a work permit they are tested for Aids and STD's before they start to work. They pay daily for the room and the rest is all theirs.

Campo is definitely a place worth visiting. It is one of the best values in the world. The going rate is only 50 Guilders or roughly $28 for about half an hour. Some of the girls are really hot and on par with the high-class hookers you get in other parts of the world. Guaranteed you will receive better service than most high class call girls.

In many of the Islands you will find working girls at strip joints. In Curacao, this was a legal way around the law for having a whorehouse. The entertainment permit states for "any entertainment". The girls are given temporary work permits as dancers. If a local person does not desire a certain position, a foreigner may apply. Nearly all the working girls come from other countries or Islands.

In Aruba these places are mostly restricted to an area called Saint Nicholas. This is a bit of a drive from the city of Oranjestad. The average price in Aruba runs about $100. The working girls of the islands typically do the circuit of Curacao, Aruba and Saint Martin. They spend three months at each place before going home to relax few a few months or weeks.

Other locations in Saint Maarten are Carolinas which mostly has Colombian, Dominican, Jamaican women. Golden Eye, a Strip Club, mostly had eastern block and Turkish women. Defiance Haven had eastern bloc, European, Colombian and Dominican woman. Le Petite Chateau predominately had West Indian, Colombian and Venezuelan women. Carmen Priest also known as Sunset Retreat had mostly Colombian and Dominican women. Crystal Club was frequented by Venezuelan women. Platinum Room, a classy Strip Cub with an indoor pool, had European, Eastern Block, Jamaican, Venezuelan and women from the British Virgin Islands. Bada Bing a Strip Club next to the airport runway, you will find Eastern Block and Dutch women.

Another place that has made its mark is Panama, with many of the Colombians including this destination in their hooking itinerary. Nevertheless, the price is steep as the local currency is US Dollars. It can end costing you $100 just to take the girl out of the clubs and $ 250 for the girl. Though there are places you can find that will only cost you $100.

CAMPO ALEGRE

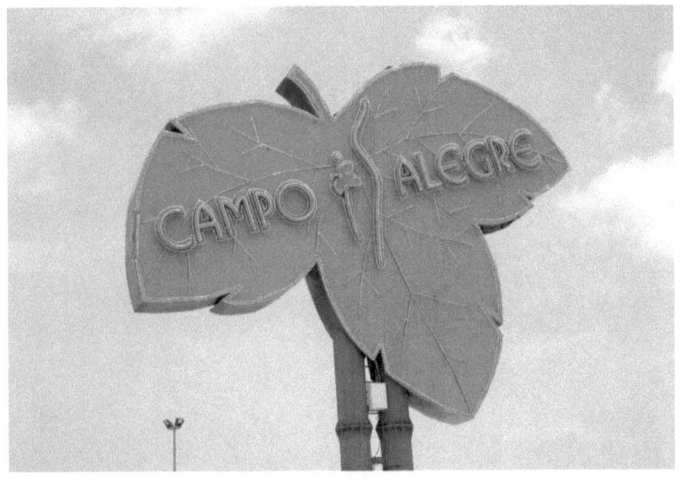

the sign

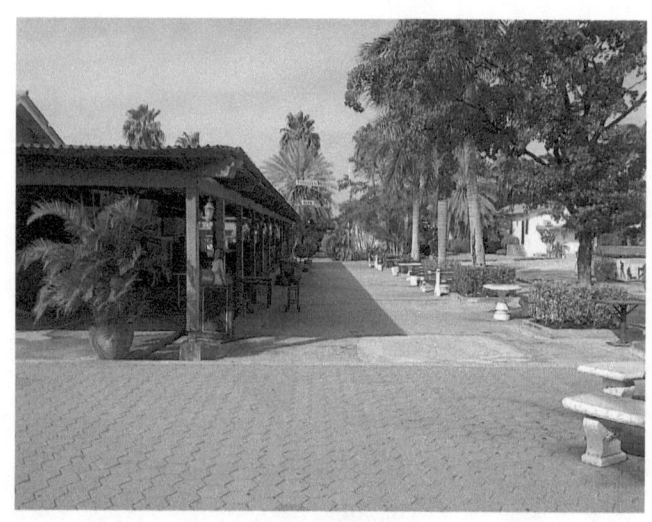

bar area

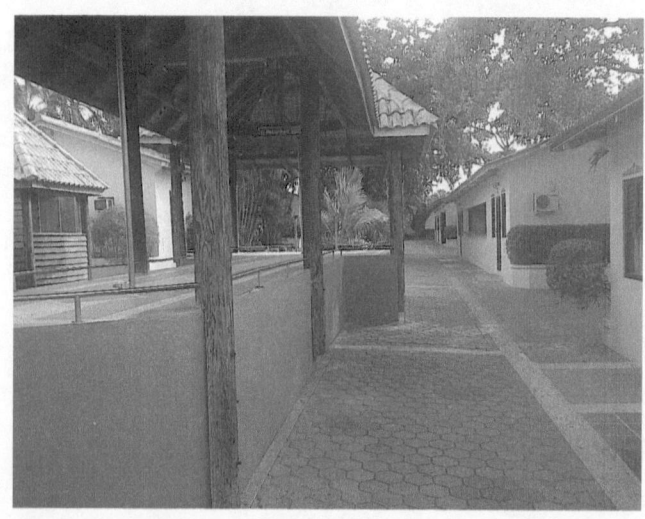

outdoor stage

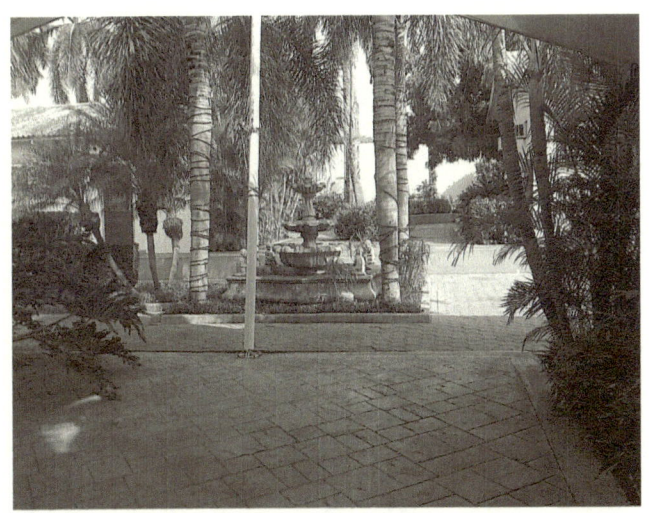

a Fountain

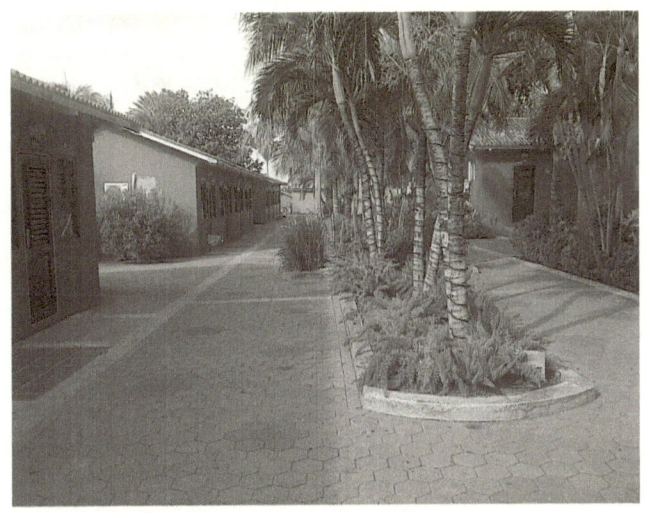

rows of rooms

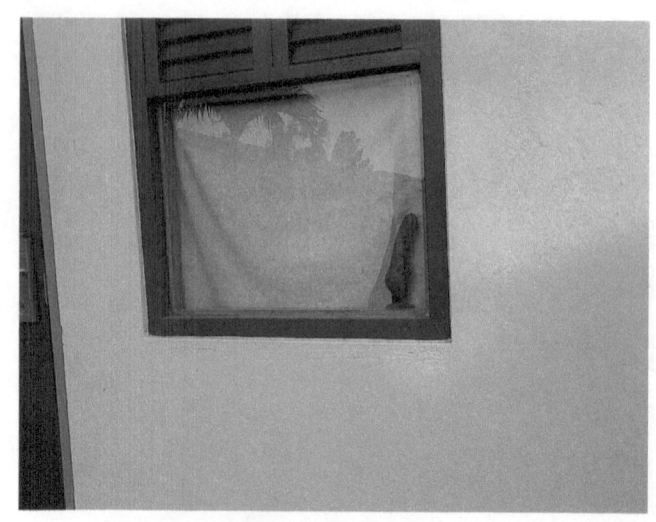

window display

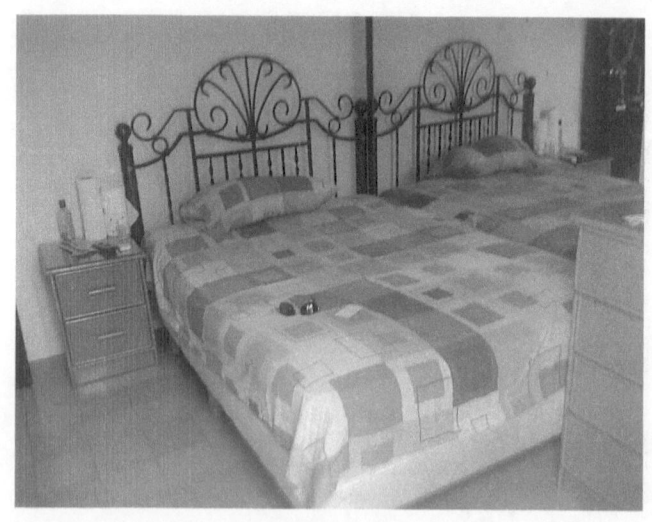

inside a room

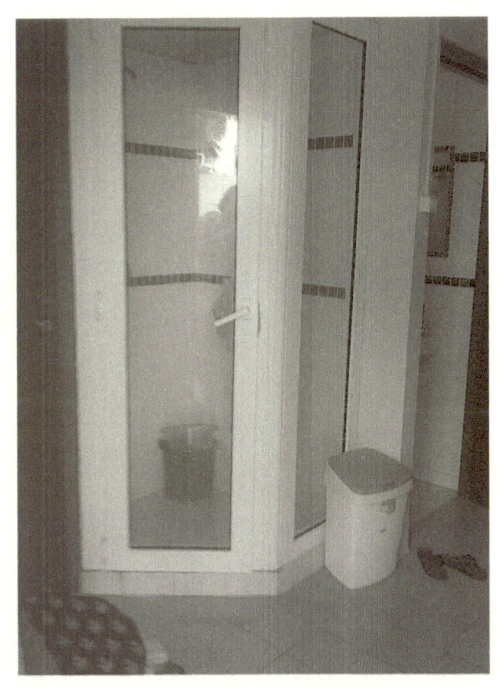

a shower in a room

CHAPTER 3
WHO, WHY, HOW

This question has intrigued many men and some women for ages. Why do some women venture into the life of prostitution? A simple answer would be some for financial reasons and some out of pure fascination. Others get into the profession for the basic reason that they are born to be whores. They actually enjoy the sex and money. A married British woman made a comment during an interview that she felt she was born to be a whore. Her husband approved of her chosen profession and even joined in at times. In Latin America due to the lack of employment for women it is the best option available for young pretty girls. Some have made it a career and retired at the ripe age of 40 with houses paid for and business set up in their home countries. Here are some girls I met along the way and their reasons for getting into the business.

Adriana

Age: 24

Nationality: Colombian

Vital statistics: 5'6", long dark hair, average body, size C tits

She was one of the kinkiest nymphs I have ever met. As she hadn't had any children she had a fairly tight pussy, but had loosened a little, having been fucked so much. When only 15yrs old she encountered an elderly man while walking home from school one day. He called her over and offered her large amount of money to have sex with him. She was impressed by the amount of money she was offered and made the decision to oblige. Unexpectedly he fucked her in the ass, which she said was extremely painful. Still, even after that experience, she said she found her true calling in life. Ever since that day she would fuck, suck, take it up the ass, and swallow for any amount of money. I have never met a woman who enjoys sex as she does. She told me she was not money crazy like most working girls, but fucked and sucked out of pure enjoyment. With this attitude in mind, she ended up making more money than most women. Many customers would pay her more than the going rate as she gave such excellent service. You will read further stories about her later in this book.

Lisa
Age: 26
Nationality: Colombian
Vital Statistics: 5'8", long brown hair, average body, size A tits (she wished to get a boob job in order to make her hotter), smooth shaved pussy with no protruding lips, only the slit visible

She had been divorced by the age of 22. She had been left without money to fend for herself and her three children after her divorce. Her sister suggested to her to go to Curacao to work as a whore at Campo Alegre. She helped her arrange flights and all the other necessary arrangements to go to Curacao. She sat in her room the first day at Campo crying while men waited outside her door to try her out. A friend had suggested she get high on Marijuana, which she did. It seemed to help her get over the first initial customers. Soon she learned to enjoy it and indulged in her client's fantasies with enthusiasm.

Luz
Age: 24
Nationality: Colombian
Vital Statistics: 5'6", natural blond, curvy body, fairly tight pussy

One of the most honest, down to earth whores I have ever met. She had a distinctive scar across her chest and stomach diagonally. I never bothered to ask her what had caused that. She started fucking for money when she was young as it felt the most natural thing to do. Even back home, she would work as a whore in the local tavern. Some women claim that they would never work as a whore back home or will let family members know what work they did. She admitted that she was a whore and one of the few whores who would thank you for fucking her afterwards, knowing well that the funds would help the family back home.

Patricia
Age: 29
Nationality: Colombian
Vital statistics: 5'5", shoulder length blond hair, hot body and pert tits

She got into the game for pure financial gain. She was married, but her husband had no problem with her traveling and applying her trade. She owned houses and taxi's back home. This girl had applied her trade in a professional and friendly way. Never saw her after a while, so I can only assume after years of working she must have finally hung up her condoms.

Lucia, Adriana & Lucy all in their early 20's. Lucia and Adriana were half sisters and Lucy their cousin. They were family members who decided to travel to the Islands to make some money for Christmas. Lucy and Adriana told their families they were working in hotels, while Lucia said she worked in an electronic store. She even took pictures of herself in front of a local electronic store to show her parents. Little did their parents know that the work they did was either on their backs, kneeling down or sitting on their clients, fucking to their hearts content. All three girls were hot and into some lesbian fun. What a turn on to see two cousins or sisters having ago at each other.

Sandra
Age: 39
Nationality: Colombian
Vital Statistics: tall athletic body, still very hot for her age, some obvious plastic surgery

She was well educated and fluent in English. She read thick English novels. She was what you called a career prostitute. She started about 18 years old purely for the financial gain. Sandra was a straightforward woman. Would not even leave the whorehouse in the daytime, knowing that she was there to fuck for money and time was money. She was in the final phase of her career. As she had said, she had paid for her house through her pussy, ass and mouth. She was now saving money to buy a house for her mother. Afterwards . . . . retirement. How many people do you know that can say they can retire at the age of 39, even though it was after 21 years of fucking?

Isabel
Age: late 40' or early 50's
Vital statistics: 5'5", long brown hair, good body, size C tits

Was one of the oldest whores I have ever met in Curacao. Already in her late 40's or early 50's when I first met her. Although I cannot say much about her face, she still got plenty of work. She had started in the business in her early twenties for financial reasons. Occasionally she would travel to other Islands to apply her trade. Over the years she was able to open up her own successful clothing boutique in her hometown. Probably the longest working whore I ever met, almost 30 years of sex for money. At an average of working 6 months a year for 30 years, she had about over 1.2km of cocks that have been in her pussy.

Carmen
Age: 19
Nationality: Dominican Republic
Vital Statistics: 5'5", shoulder length dark hair, slightly oriental look, perfect little body, small firm tits

Carmen came to the island to work as a barmaid at a local strip club. She was very pretty and often had offers made to her over the counter. It did not take her long to figure out that there was more money to be made on the other side of the counter. You will read an interesting story about her later in the book.

Alejandra
Age: 26
Nationality: Colombian
Vital Statistics: Petite blond, size C tits, and tight pussy

She came from a very poor family in Colombia. At the age of 18 she realized that she wanted some of the finer things of life. She took a hard look at her life and finally made the difficult decision to go into prostitution. Panama was where she headed to start her new profession. 8 years later she is still hard at work, and indeed enjoying the finer things in life with the help of her pussy. At that moment she had no intention to settle down and marry. She worked with a lot of passion, and one of the few women who would allow you to kiss her on the mouth if she fancies you. A very pleasant person, one you would gladly take home to meet your mother.

Martha
Age: 19
Nationality: Colombian
Vital Statistics: petite, long straight dark hair, large breasts, tight pussy

One of the few girls I have met whose parents know what she is up to and approve of her doing the work. She got into the business to help her poor parents. She is a pleasant girl who loves her work. Demanding that her customers *"duro Papi duro"* which means "fuck me hard Papi" *Pap*i is a term most Latin women use to lovingly call their man. I had first thought it had to do with a strange incestuous obsession they had with their fathers.

Carolina
Age: 29
Vital Statistics: beautiful strange slender body that could resemble a native na'vi woman from the movie Avatar, pretty face, long blond hair

Carolina was friendly and well-educated. She had only to finish one more year at University to obtain her degree in Accounting. She spoke fluent English. She remarked one day that after leaving Campo she would do "three" months in Aruba, and another "three" months in St. Maarten. Then it will be off to university to finish her degree and no more "fucky

fucky, sucky sucky". She wanted a more professional job as an accountant. Of course I think experience counting money could be added to her resume. In one hour I had observed three satisfied clients. After she was finished servicing a customer, condom in hand she would look at it and say "hello babies", and then say "good bye babies" as she would dispose of the condom in the garbage. A friend of mine once said it was worth just paying her to see her naked body.

The most common story I hear about many of these women is they met a man while quite young. They have a child together and then the man abandons them. The woman is left alone to take care of herself and their children. Typically as they are very young at the time, they lack both education and experience. Jobs are limited and the pay is poor for unskilled laborers. The most natural job they can get is to open their legs and make some money.

I have come across a lot of University students who travel on their breaks to work as hookers to collect tuition money. I met two well-educated Colombian women once at Campo who were hot and had athletic bodies. Both enjoyed collecting their tuition funds and having sexual fun. Some would even take off for a whole year to travel around the Caribbean to earn the money. This is now becoming a popular choice in other parts of the world for students to pay for their studies. In the USA and UK these female students are referred to as a "sugar babies"

There are also "part-time" working girls from all kinds of backgrounds or situations. Like **Sandra,** a barmaid, who was married. She would have non-negotiable price of Naf.100 ($55) for her services. Her husband did not mind as it would bring extra cash for them. She had long brown hair, pretty face and voluptuous body. She would not seek out her clients, but if a customer from the bar or restaurant she worked at happened to ask her for sex, she would oblige. She would go home with them or to a hotel at the end of her shift. Unfortunately the last I heard of her was that she was serving jail time in Colombia for theft.

Pamela
Age: late 20's
Nationality: Colombian
Vital Statistics: A lovely Julia Roberts look alike

She did some part-time administration work and had the best way of putting things. She would say she was not a "puta", but if a man wants to help her pay the rent, then she would have sex with him to show her appreciation.

Another part time working girl was **Helen** who worked in a hotel. She was a slim Venezuelan woman with a child. If she had a high phone or utility bill to pay, she would spread her legs to collect the money. At a time she had a phone bill of about $200 to pay, so she was prepared to offer two hours of sex with anyone will to pay the bill.

In Caracas, Venezuela in the early 90's I came across a bar that had the most beautiful women I have ever seen. I was visiting Caracas with my wife at the time. It was still early in the evening when I entered the bar first, my wife just a step behind me. As I walked in I noticed all the beautiful women stare at me and could hear them utter "yeeeh!" but as soon as they saw my wife they uttered "aaaah". I must have been among the first few men to walk through the door that evening. After we ordered drinks the women were not afraid to approach us. Turned out most of the girls were varsity students. They would come to the bar to use their pussies to pay for their tuition. Almost all of these women were like models or Miss Venezuela. Classy and beautiful. The going rate for these women back then was $100. This was a justified price for the quality of these women.

There are married women who do resort to prostitution, mostly with their husbands consent. Some of them do it full time, part-time or when the opportunity arises. I knew of a Dutchmen whose wife was Colombian. She had blond hair (obliviously not natural) and a well proportioned body. She would hire herself out as a companion to men visiting the island.

Sometimes for a few days or a full week. Another couple was also a slim Colombian woman who had a local "island" husband. She mostly catered to the expats or foreigners on the Island. You would arrive at their house, which was located a bit out of the way, and the husband would greet you at the door. He'd then invite you into the living room to wait for his wife. The wife soon appeared after taking a shower. Her hair still wet, she was fresh and clean, ready for action. She would then lead you to a vacant room to perform her services while her husband watched TV in the lounge. I wondered if he had a camera in the room, so he could watch live while his wife was fucked by a client. This was normally her day job as she was a dancer at one of the local strip joints in the evening.

A movie that gives you a good deal of insight into some of the backgrounds of these women and the choices they make is "Maria Full of Grace". About a young Colombian woman who decides to escape from her poverty by becoming a drug mule. Unlike Maria who swallows Cocaine *"Bolitas"*, these girls opt to use their pussies to make money. I have never been to Colombia, but after seeing this movie, it gave me a better idea about the lives of the Colombian women I have met that explained their hardships they endured before going into prostitution. The actress Catalina Sandino Moreno was nominated for her role for an Academy Award in 2005.

I came across a beautiful woman once who came to work at Campo out of necessity. She was from Colombia, tall with a slight oriental look. I don't know if she either did not know what the work actually entailed or she learned the hard way that this was not the work for her. She might have thought she was just there to dance as she did take part in the nightly strip show. After just one week of work she packed up and went home.

Of the three groups of why the girls get into the business: love to fuck, financial, no other option; I would say that I have met plenty of women who fall into the first category. I have to say all of them are in it for financial reasons. I don't really buy the reason that they have no option but to fuck for money. Some uneducated girls opt to be maids or cleaners. Many of them are pretty enough to make money with their pussies. Each made their choices, morally or otherwise.

CHAPTER 4
THE BACHELOR PARTIES

There is nothing better than a group of horny guys getting together with some booze and hot Latino women. It sure makes for a good combination and some interesting scenarios.

It was some time in the 1990's that a friend of ours Greg was getting married. We decided to throw him a surprise bachelor party. The fun began when Robert, Bart and I set out a week before to find some willing girls to join in the festivities.

It was a Wednesday night and we set out to La Tasca, a local nightclub where working girls go to pick up clients. La Tasca commonly known as LT's, was located just off a main street in the downtown area of Otrabanda in Curacao. In the earlier years it was a well known place to go if you wanted a "Take Away". The girls were not bound to the premises as they are in some other places. These women were freelance hookers. There were two hotels on the same street where most of the girls stayed, the Park Hotel and Hotel Carlos. The going rate at that time for the women was about $55 (Fls.100) and an additional $6 for the room, even though the girl had already rented the room. A nice additional income for the hotel owners or receptionist as I am sure some of them would have pocketed the money for themselves. There was always a good mixture of girls, mainly Dominicans, Colombians, Venezuelans and Jamaicans.

I remember a time I did not bother to get a room and decided to settle for a blowjob in the car park. I relaxed in the driver's seat as her head bobbed up and down on my dick. I looked up to make sure no one was watching and saw the security guard in the distance slowly making his way towards us. I knew I had to cum before he reached my car. "Suck harder" I explained to the woman in Spanish knowing I had just a few minutes before he would reach me. When he was just about 20 meters away, I exploded as I pushed her head down. It was just in time for her to remove the condom, wipe her mouth and for me to zip up as the security guard passed by.

Anyway, we entered the bar about 9pm. Typically the place would only start to get going about 10pm. The place was full with well-dressed women. I remember bringing an American female friend to the place without telling her what kind of a place it was. She was dressed in jeans. We sat down and ordered some beers. After looking around she commented to me that she felt a little under dressed for the place and that the women were all dressed in formal attire. I later let her in on to what kind of place it was. She took it in a good spirit, even commenting on some of the women's beauty.

We started talking to some girls and soon found two girls who were willing to do a lesbian show. They were not all that hot, but we took their telephone numbers, names and told them we would pick them up the following week. Then I ran into a girl I had met there before. Jackie was not that good looking but had a heart of gold. She was interested in getting in on the action. I offered her the job of topless barmaid, which she accepted. She would later on be always known as the "Ugly One". To be fair to her she was not that bad. Nevertheless, compared to the other girls who were at the party she was the least pretty.

Next we decided to head off to one of my old favorite places, Stellaris. This was an old hotel located just down the street from LT's overlooking the harbor entrance. There was a seedy bar located at the back of the hotel that was dark, but gave you a sense of privacy.

This was primarily a place with Colombian and Dominican girls. There was a time when a group of Brazilian girls were staying there. They ended up pissing off the other Latino girls as they came in and under cut them. They were charging a bit less for a fuck. I have to say Brazilian girls do know how to fuck. The going rate was only about $42 and you did not have to pay for the room.

Stellaris was an old building with wooden floors, so when you walked to the bar in the back you would hear the floors creak. To enter the bar you had to pass through the hotel entrance down a dark passage way and then make a right turn past the male toilets. Then turn left down another short passage and enter through a doorway facing the ladies toilet with a dance floor in front of you. To your right was a large L shaped bar about 10 paces back, table and chairs spread out over the comfortable size room. We entered the low lit bar, looked around and saw a fair selection of woman. By this time we had quite a few drinks under our belt. Consequently the woman looked a lot prettier than the LT girls.

I saw a tall beautiful woman sitting legs crossed at the bar. I walked up to her and was greeted by a smile. Her name was Lucia. I looked into her beautiful green eyes and felt an immediate connection. I later found out that the green eyes were just color contacts hiding her dark brown eyes. This is where we met the two sisters and cousin mentioned previously. Lucia and Lucy, the cousins, were interested in doing the lesbian show. They both looked a lot better than the other two we had previously signed up. So now we had to think of a way to dump the other two.

Then we met their friend Belinda, a wild voluptuous girl with long dark hair. We asked her what she could bring to the party. She replied with a classic answer, "I will go around and suck the guys' cocks while the show is on". "You're hired!" was my immediate response.

Finally the night arrived. The house was free of kids and wives. We held the party indoors in an open concept spacious living room and dining room with tiled floors, common in the Caribbean. The bar was located in the corner, well stocked with Amstel lager and White Label Scotch whisky. All curtains and blinds closed and air conditioner set high. A space blanket that I had used during my European backpacking days was laid out on the floor, ready for the girl on girl show as oil was to be used.

Bart picked up the girls from their hotel. All women dressed for the occasion in sexy dresses and high heels. Their goal was to look hot and try to make money. Lucia looked stunning in a sexy red dress, strappy high heel shoes, and the green colored contact lenses. A face worthy of being a model or girl next door porn star. When Jackie arrived she immediately took off her top and bra and went straight to work behind the bar, exposing her firm large boobs. All the men had arrived and were just waiting for Greg to show up. We had told him we were having a barbeque so he must bring drinks and meat. He arrived with a six-pack in one hand and meat in the other. We said to him "Sorry there is no barbeque today". He looked a bit confused.

Then we led him in and the party began. Let me tell you, what a party it turned out to be.

With all the guys present and with drinks in hand, Lucia and Lucy approached each other. Slow sultry music playing and they moved their sexy bodies to the music. Both had long dark hair. Lucia was the taller one with the attractive green eyes. Lucy was shorter but had a good curvy body. Anticipation could be felt in the room the closer they got to each other. The temperature was rising and energy in the air. When they were just inches away from each other, their lips slowly parted and they finally connected. Tongues engaged, caressing and lovingly. As they continued the heated kissing they started to undress one another. Dresses fell to the floor, revealing their sexy bodies.

While standing naked together they rubbed breasts against one another. Their hands caressed each others' face, breasts, arms and running down the length of the back to each others' ass. One of the girls reached for a bottle of beautiful sensually scented oil. Slowly they massaged a generous amount all over each other's bodies. Their beautiful olive skinned bodies glistering in the light. They dropped down on the space blanket. Now laying down they writhed together, bodies entwined, this time to the song of "Stairway to Heaven". At this time we all realized we were in heaven. Lucia spread her cousin's legs, tongue exploring her pussy, parting her lips and entering into her wet pussy with her tongue. Skillfully she worked her tongue towards the clitoris, massaging it in a flicking motion. Lucy laid back legs apart groaning in ecstasy. All men's eyes glued to this beautiful display of womanly love. We also forgot all about that at this time Belinda was suppose to go around sucking cocks while Lucia and Lucy were in incestuous passion. Instead she sat next to Mark stroking his cock through his pants.

By the end of the show doors were opening and men and woman were disappearing into the bedrooms and even the bathroom. The fucking had begun. There was a teenage guy name Ronnie who was borrowing money from everyone, as he was on a rampage to fuck all the women. Guys were getting blow jobs in the lounge. Guys were banging on doors so they could get a room.

At this time, the only woman who was not getting fucked was the "Ugly One". So Juan Carlos grabbed her by the hand and led her to my bedroom, which was out of limits to the rest of the guys and asked me if I wanted to join in. They entered in the room and I joined them a few minutes later. As I entered, I saw Juan Carlos had the "Ugly One" on all fours doggie style. His cock was ramming away into her wet hairy pussy. At this stage, I walked over and stood in front of her as she was just on the edge of the bed. I undid my pants and inserted my cock into her mouth. "Awe this is good" explained Juan Carlos grabbing her by the hair and forcing her head onto my cock, almost causing her to choke. Nevertheless, I could see Jackie was enjoying this. As she sucked hard on my cock I looked up to see Juan Carlos wiping away the sweat on his forehead grinning as he pumped her harder and harder. I could see he was thoroughly enjoying this. It was difficult for me to cum my load. So I left Juan Carlos to finish her off, as he continued to ram away from behind.

All the girls ended up being fucked about three to four times each, making it a worthwhile adventure for them. A few years later, we arranged another show. We bumped into the "Ugly One" again and invited to the show. This time she appeared to have improved her looks a bit, even shaving her pussy and flashing it during the show. She turned out to be the most fun girl at the party and gave the best service that night.

Another bachelor party of note was "The Missing Clock party", which it later became remembered by. It involved an Englishman, a visiting mad Englishman, Portuguese (the Bachelor), Venezuelan, Australian and some South Africans. They had arranged a private lesbian show with two women, in one of their rooms at Campo. One of these women was a wild woman, who was later referred to as the "Biter", as she would bite you as you are having sex with her.

The show involved two women going at each other, licking each other and ramming dildos up their sweet pussies. Afterwards they pulled one of the men onto the bed and began to service him. A few of us had noticed a clock in the room, which Juan Carlos had later stated the time on the clock was wrong.

After the show Juan Carlos and I had sat down at the bar to have a few more drinks. Everyone else had left at that point. A security guard approached us with one of the girls from the show. She pointed at us, and said that we were the ones. The security guards are known in Campo as the "Watchyman". He made us stand up and we were searched. We asked what was going on in. The Watchyman replied explaining that someone had stolen the girl's clock. This was a strange item to be stolen as an item for memorabilia. You'd think it would have been panties. Still to this day it remains a mystery. Who had taken the clock and why? We all assumed that either the mad Englishman or the Venezuelan had taken it.

There was a painful Bachelor party one night, where the stripper accidently stood on Ken's balls. He lay beneath her as she danced over him flashing her shaved pussy while gyrating. I was not present at this party, but was told that besides the painful balls, it was a pleasurable night.

My Bachelor party was at Copacabana, the strip place that opened at 12am and carried on until 6am. My best man treated me to a lovely 18-year-old Dominican dancer. She spent the whole night with me, well what was left of the night. I ended up only having one hour sleep before going off to work.

I must say that I have been one of the few married man who has had their wife arrange "special birthday party". My wife and friend Bob had arranged a hot Colombian woman named Danielle to dance for me. I was a bit embarrassed hand cuffed to the chair with her dancing around me. So I suggested we finish off the show in the room. My wife armed with a video camera filmed the whole event as I was able to finish off the show fucking her hard in my bedroom.

Danielle was a beautiful woman with long dark silky hair and great personality. One I would call marriage material. Soon after that I never saw her working again, which I am sure some lucky man had scooped her up and made her his permanent fuck. At least I still have the video I can watch when I am an old man reminiscing about my youth.

In 2003 I attended a bachelor party for a friend in St Maarten. There were about 20 guys at Jack's party. Nigel, the organizer, had hired a bus for the night. The night started off visiting regular bars and a dinner at some restaurant, where Jack's brother sang with the band "You can't always get what you want".

Nigel had promised Jack's future wife that he will not take the party to any Strip places or whorehouses. Nigel had stuck to his guns until we managed to get him to change plans, even with Jack's blessing.

First stop was the Platinum Room, a classy place with mostly Russian girls. The place had an indoor pool in front of the stage. As soon as the girls heard it was a bachelor party, they were delighted to take Jack up on the stage. They danced and stripped around him as he sat on a chair stripped down to his underpants. After they pulled him into the pool and lay him on a floating mattress. A beautiful Russian girl was rubbing her wet pussy in his face. I have the photos on file as I was the unofficial photographer for the night.

We ended the night at some whorehouse up on a hill. At the bar I met a sexy blond Colombian woman. She was wearing thigh high boots. We soon ended up in her room. I asked her if I can take some photos of her and she gladly agreed. She gave me all different posses spreading her legs revealing her clean pussy and ass. I could not cum though due to my drunken state. So I decided to take her back to my hotel room. The guys were a bit pissed off as they were waiting at the bus, but after seeing the hot take-a-way, it calmed them down. I had excellent service that night. She allowed me to cum all over her smooth white stomach. Sadly the pictures taken her in her room were not the best, probably because the photographer (me) was so drunk at the time. Still, I did record the moment. Anyway I met up with her again in Campo a few months later, still wearing her boots. I was turned off her this time as she snorted coke in front of me before giving service. If a woman decides to use drugs, that is her prerogative, but don't do it in front of a client. A few years later I saw her in a porno video clip on the internet, wearing her boots once again.

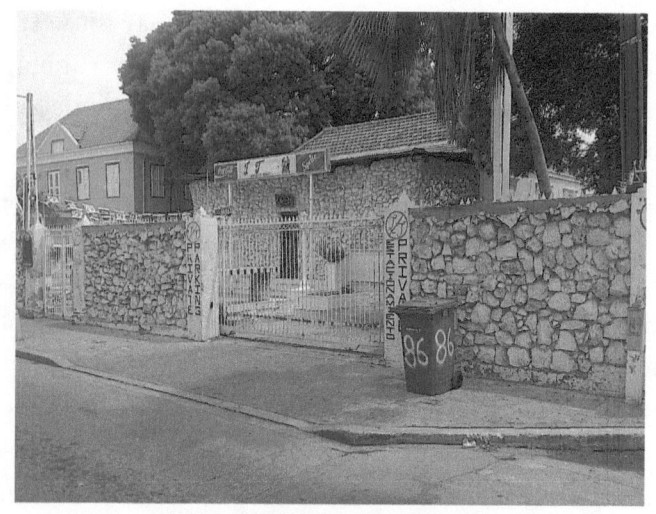

La Tasca, Curacao

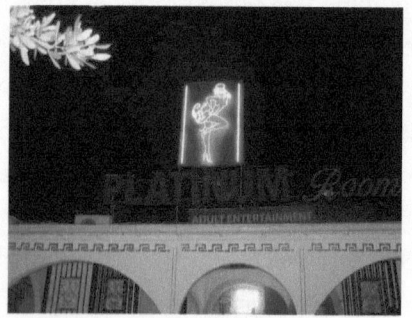

Platinum Room, St Maarten

CHAPTER 5

TOUGH WORK

Many girls enjoy their work while others just tolerate it. At times it's fun, adventurous and stimulating, but other times it can be tough work. When the going gets tough they are able to somehow switch off their consciousness and perform their services without guilt or shame.

An ex-hooker once explained to me that she would switch off her brain and perform in a Zombie like state. Some use Cocaine or Marijuana to help them switch off or numb their minds. An escape from reality. It can be a tough job but someone is always willing to do it.

At Campo, the women have to pay $50 per day for the room. They must also pay for their own flights to Curacao, food and condoms. That means they must service at least two customers just to pay for the room. For those less attractive slow times could be hard on them. If they participate in the show they get a discount on the room. At the bar they have a closed in show room with a stage and stripper pole. Large screen TV's showing porno movies or sports. There are daily strip shows, which can include a sex show with two women or a male participant from the audience.

Lisa had one of her better nights at Campo. She took on 13 customers in an 8-hour period. Her body eventually took strain. She had to fuck a lot in doggy style, her torso taking a beating from been pumped from behind. Eventually she just had to close her door, as she could not take any more. Nevertheless, with no regrets as it was a very profitable night for her making over $400 for just 8 hours work. As mentioned before Campo has about the best rates in the world, as the basic going rate is only $28.

A few weeks later I ran into Lisa again, she had gone one better. There were only a few girls working at Campo at that time, as there was a delay in the work permits for the new batch of girls. She had started fucking from 4pm in the afternoon and continued until 10am the next morning. She managed to service 18 clients the whole night, a new record for her. As one client left her room, the next was waiting outside for his turn.

I met a Colombian divorcee who kept her hourglass figure by regular working out in a gym. She claimed to have had 30 men in one day. She had been married to a wealthy man who used to use drugs and beat her up. She managed to divorce him and getting custody of their two children. Now she has her freedom traveling, working as a hooker, while her family takes care of her kids.

The two students I mentioned before had a good run one week. They purchased a bag of 100 condoms between the two of them. The whole bag only lasted 4 days, making it a tough but profitable 4 days. That is about 50 men each in 4 days. As I mentioned before, these two girls really enjoyed the work even when the going gets tough.

Another Adriana II had a customer in the room for over an hour, resulting in men pacing up and down outside her room waiting their turn. Turned out she had one of her regular customers who had such a thick cock, that she was unable to put it into her mouth. She would have to just lick around the head to arouse him. Once his cock was hard, lying on her back she would spread her legs and ever so slowly let him gently insert his cock. Only being able to handle just a few strokes she would pull it out to let her pussy relax. Then have another go at it, this procedure lasting over an hour until he exploded. It never crossed my mind at the time to ask her if she had special size condoms for this client.

I had a temporary maid at my home in the early 1990's. Maria was in her early thirties and not a bad body back then. She wore jeans pretty well, and had nice firm tits. Maria would work for us during the day, then dress up at night and hit the bars or hotels in search of customers. One morning she returned in a bit of pain, walking with her legs slightly apart and back bent. She told us that she had a man with such a long cock that it hurt the back of her pussy and also gave her back pain. The next night she rested her pussy, as this was the longest dick she had ever taken all the way. Most women place their hands on the man's stomach acting as a restraint, to prevent full penetration and allowing the amount of penetration they can handle.

Another Maria, an older street hooker, said her toughest one was a customer whose dick stunk to high heaven. He would make her suck his cock and she would have to hold in to avoid throwing up. I don't know why she didn't just wash it before sucking. Most of the Campo girls give you a refreshing feminine hygiene soap they use to clean their pussies. The soap leaves your cock and balls feeling fresh and cool, ready to put it between parted lips as their tongue massages under your helmet.

Probably the hardest part of the job is when the girls are new to anal sex. Plenty complain that it is extremely painfully the first few times. However, as time goes by and about 50 cocks later they say it loosens up. Not all girls allow anal as they say it is too painful to try. However, Adriana mentioned in Chapter 3 said her first time with the older man when she was a schoolgirl was excruciating. Now she loves it finding the need to use two dildos on herself when times are quiet, one in each hole.

I met a Doctor who had worked in the local hospital in the emergency ward. There have been quite a few cases of women been rushed to the hospital from Campo with objects either stuck up their ass or pussies. You would be amazed at what objects had to be removed. Everything from bath sponges, deodorant caps, condoms, broken dildos, candles, panties, bottles etc . . . . When a bottle is used as a sex toy without the cap on, a vacuum is created from being stroked up and down. This suction action results with the bottle getting stuck up there. So remember ladies if you want to insert a bottle up your pussy, remember to leave the cap on. It must be quite an embarrassing experience for these women. It would not surprise me if some male customers were rushed to the hospital for similar problems.

Lucia had a customer who had the same kinky request each time he would visit her. He would bend over on all fours and wait for his strange desire. Then with her hand and arm well lubricated, she would slowly insert her fingers up his ass. Eventually she inserted her whole hand and pushing deeper almost reaching her elbow. Lucia was quite a tall woman so it was quite a deep insertion. Then she would stroke his dick with the other hand and he would rapidly cum his load. I have heard of girls sticking their fingers up the guys' asses, but the whole arm takes the cake.

Lucia, her sister and cousin once invited me for dinner in their room one evening at Stellaris. The three of them shared a room with three beds. Cooking in the rooms was not permitted. However, it was amazing the meal they managed to cook, using only a rice cooker. The meal was a typical Latin meal of rice, beans and meat. Hopefully they cleaned her hands before cooking!

Some women do not enjoy the work and explain that they have no other options. When I asked one of these girls what it was like to have to work if she did not enjoy what she was doing. She explained it to me in the most simple and understanding way, "Imagine you have to allow men to fuck you up the ass so you can feed your children". You have to do what you have to do. I must say it was a painful thought.

Copacabana was a nightclub hidden off the beaten track on a street called Roseveltweg in Curacao. It was home to mostly Jamaican strippers and hookers, and a few Dominicans. The Jamaican women had very different style of dancing. They would do handstands back towards the wall, with their legs against the wall. They would gyrate their bodies to the music, swirling their hips around. Each table was fitted with a bicycle bell in the center of the table, so you could ring for service. A friend of mine Tony use to love going to this place as he would fall asleep for a while then wake up to watch the show bit. Then sleep for a while more and so on. The shows would only start at about 12am and carry on until sunrise. We spent plenty nights there for the full 6 hours.

Rick and I had decided to go over to Copacabana earlier in the evening to see what women were available. A pretty Dominican woman was working behind the bar. She was the only woman available at that time. We decided to share her and take her back to her room, which was located at the back. We each had our turn fucking her while the other would get a blowjob. Rick and I were new to this kind of threesome and found the scenario difficult to make us cum. For over an hour we fucked this poor woman, who was enjoying it at first, as this was also a new exciting experience for her taking on two guys at once. Eventually she started begging us to stop saying *"no mas, no mas porfavor"*. No more, no more please. We told her that we needed to cum. Eventually I came up with the idea of waiting by the bathroom out of view, while Rick finished off. Then he went out of view while I finished off. The poor girl had just been fucked constantly for almost two hours solid.

Many women that I spoke to claim they are only in it for the money and who claim not to enjoy the work. They say that it is tough having their bodies touched all over and having to change sexual positions a lot. Most of these women use drugs or alcohol to block out their senses of reality.

In 2008 I was surprised to see something in the same month in two different parts of the world. I came across pregnant working girls. The first two I saw was at a disco in a Casino in Sosua, Dominican Republic. The Government had changed the law that after 1 am no alcohol can be sold, but fortunately for the Casino this law did not apply. Around 1 am their disco would fill up with all the hookers in the area. I sat at the bar observing all different types and styles of "working girls" entering the disco. I counted over 60 women entering the nightclub. To my surprise there were two pregnant women dressed up sexy, bellies protruding. They were there to see if they can make some money. There are men who have the fetish desire to fuck a pregnant woman.

A few days later I flew to Canada where I visited one of the strip joints in Niagara Falls. There is a street called Lundy's Lane, a short drive from the main Niagara Falls center. The first place I went to had plenty of women. The second woman to get up and dance was the pregnant one. She was a tall, long brown hair, pretty face. She spun around the pole spreading her legs. I had a humorous thought of seeing a small hand coming out her pussy waving to the crowd has she spread her beautiful long legs. Have to say Canadian woman are great. No attitudes like some of the women you find in other parts of the world.

I did put one to test, not the pregnant one, but one of the other sexy Canadian girls. I asked her if she is allowed to make a guy cum during a lap dance. Politely she replied "yes". On my third lap dance she straddled me naked rubbing her pussy against my cock. She had placed a small towel on my lap at the start of the lap dance. With one hand playing with my balls, the other squeezing the end of my cock, she rode me hard. It did not take too long into the song before I came in my pants. A lap dance costs $20, but it was so good I gave her an extra $20 for the pleasure. I could see that she enjoyed it as well. I was a little bit embarrassed as I left the area because I had a big wet patch in my pants. I tried to cover with my shirt. With the low lights, probably no one noticed it.

CHAPTER 6

EASY MONEY

There are times when the girls say they have it easy. They don't have to do too much work or make a lot of effort to make the money.

The customers that Lucia said she had the easiest times with were the Korean Seaman from the ships. The ships would dock on the Otrabanda side of the harbor of Curacao. It's just a short walk up the hill to Hotel Stellaris. Lucia would either go back to the ship with them or take them to her hotel room which she shared with her sister and cousin. She would undress them and then undress herself. They would sit on the bed staring at her naked hot body. Probably noticing how very different she was from Asian women. She would then stroke their small erect cocks. In a short time they would gasp and shoot their cum straight at her. These were the fastest services she ever had to perform. It must have been either that they had not seen or been with a woman for a while or they were infatuated with non-oriental women. She noted that most of them had small cocks.

Patricia told me a similar story with some of her Oriental clients. They would grab and squeeze her breast, refuse a blowjob and as one would insert his cock into her self-lubricated pussy and drawback, they would shoot their load. Quick quick.

Another of Lucia's easy money customers was a European man from the ships. He would pay her for a full hour to be in his cabin. She would strip down naked and lie on the bed while he caressed her whole body with his hands. He would not have any type of sex with her, but instead just admire her tall well-shaped body. Lucia remarked that this was one of her most delightful working moments, to be paid by a man to give her relaxing pleasure.

I knew of an American in his late sixties who had business in Curacao. When visiting he would arrange for a woman to come to his hotel room and pay them just to eat their pussy. This was in the days before Viagra. I'd guess that probably because of his diabetic condition he may have had difficulty to get a hard on. He would pay anything from $100 to $200 for this. I am sure that the women he had must have enjoyed these encounters.

There is a term used by men frequenting Campo to describe certain working girls. They say "she is just business". These girls know that they have the looks or a great body as their main assets. They take the men into their rooms and they'd have them in and out, pardon the pun, before you know it. Pat was a short hot looking Colombian woman with long black hair. It never took her too long to pick up a customer. I would time her to see how long she would take. Typically within 15 minutes she was out again in search of her next prey.

I decided to try her just for the experience after been advised by a friend that she was "just business". Once the door closed you could sense that the clock was ticking. Stripped to just her panties she would quickly take off your clothes. Condom in hand she would start to lick your cock and before you know it, the condom is on and she is sucking you hard. Trying her best to suck and make you cum as quickly as possible. She'd attempt to talk dirty with you, and would talk as fast as possible. Surely she thought this would make you cum quicker, but I immediately got the feeling that this is all a show. A woman like this has to rely on many new customers, as I doubt she had much repeat business. After a while with experience, you learn to sense whether a woman is just business or not.

Then there are some women who try to "double" fuck you, literally and figuratively. Greg was sitting at a table with a friend at Campo when a good-looking girl approached him and asked if he was interested in a fuck or suck "*fucky, fucky, sucky, sucky*" as they would say. He remarked that he did not have money for a fuck. To his surprise, she said that it was free and that he did not have to pay for it.

Excited by this proposal he eagerly followed her to her room. Once there she instructed him to take off his clothes. He placed them on the chair and went to go wash his cock in the bathroom. After washing his cock he re-entered the room where she fulfilled the promise of a free blowjob. Satisfied by this free service he returned to the bar to order a drink. When he opened his wallet to pay for the drink he realized that he had just been "fucked". While he was in the bathroom washing his dick, she must have quickly removed the fifty guilder note that was in his wallet.

A few years ago, I had a similar experience. When I entered the room with a woman she asked me if I come there often. I mistakenly replied "no". I later realized that this was her key to rip me off, as it was only after the experience everything fell into place. She made me take off my clothes, which she folded, and carefully placed on the floor besides the bed. She instructed me to lie back on the bed with my legs hanging over the side. She kneeled down between my legs, right next to my clothes. I lay back and enjoyed the blowjob, which lasted for some time. Afterwards I opened my wallet to pay her and realized that money was missing. When I refused to pay her she called the security. She had left me just enough money in the wallet to pay for her services that the security insisted that I pay. I realized afterwards that she skillfully had been able to suck on my cock and go through my wallet at the same time.

Luckily theses woman are a small minority. Certainly the overwhelming majority will give you good value for money. It is wise to watch your wallet and try not to fall for these types of girls and their tricks.

A petite, short haired brunette named Katy had a different request one summer night while working at Campo. A friend of mine Grant was walking around when all of a sudden felt the urge to have a shit. He did not want to use the public toilet. He happened to be passing by Katy's room at the time, who he had known from a previous encounter. So he asked her if he could use the toilet in her room. While holding his stomach in desperation he offered her money in return for the favor. Fortunately she obliged. After a long while he left the room feeling relieved, thinking to himself "that shit was almost as good as a fuck". I wonder if the 20 Florin she received was worth the after smell she had to endure?

I met up with Ella once again and mentioned to her about the book I was writing. She was quick to respond "I bet you I am in the book". She was happy to hear that she had earned her a place in this book. "I have an easy money story for you" she was quick to tell me about. Just the week before she made $1900 from one generous customer. She did not want to mention what nationality this gentleman was, due to puta-client privileges. He spent the whole day with her in the room from 8am till 5pm, enjoying her company, drinking and experiencing all different kinds of fantasies.

In Amsterdam's' "Red Light" district a woman can rent a room with the famous "window" for $60 for a straight 8 hours work. They literally sit on a chair in a window for customers to see what they have on offer. These women can make up to $600 a shift starting at a rate of $60 for 15 minutes. Now with the Euro in place the going rate is about 50 Euros.

The "Red Light" district offers a large variety of women that you can find grouped in distinct sections. All around the Church you will find mostly black women. However, just venture down the alley and you find young Dutch girls. In another area there will predominantly be Thai women and in another area, transsexuals. Many of the transsexuals can easily pass for real women.

CHAPTER 7
SERVICE COUNTS

I have come across and heard of plenty of women who give excellent service. Like in any type of business, service does count. Word of mouth works in this business, as men tell another friend how good the service was he received.

Adriana is a prime example of excellent service. She would first dress up in whatever clothes you desire to see her in, prancing around the room looking sexy as ever. From her bedside table she would remove her two dildos, one for each hole. She would lie back on the bed, a dildo up her pussy and the other one up her ass. She groans with ecstasy as she gyrates with both dildos up inside herself, allowing me to take photos with my phone camera. Her pussy dripping with her juices, legs apart and knees up enjoying her dildo masturbation.

The show gets you all hot and ready for her. She licks you balls, sucking on your cock as she crouches before you. Forcing your legs apart she licks under your balls and works her tongue towards your asshole. Licking at your asshole, she forces her tongue inside, slightly penetrating you. You may fuck her in any position, penetrating her in the hole of your choice.

If you settle for just a blowjob, you can hear she takes pleasure in sucking you, groaning all the while. Touching her pussy, you feel she is wet from excitement. As she sucks you, she strokes you balls with her hand. Not pulling her head away as you cum, she takes it all in her mouth. No she does not swallow, but spits out your cum in the wash basin and rinsing your mouth with mouth wash. Adriana a true master in her profession, leaving you totally satisfied. She has no problems with you taking photos of her, even making the comment to me "you and your friends will have a good laugh over the photos".

Carmen was a blonde-haired Colombian with a voluptuous body and large firm tits. She would typically be dressed in a sexy skirt and high heels, always a smile on her face. She would give you full body massage from head to toe, taking her time ensuring your pleasure. After a satisfying massage, she then continues to fulfill your sexual desires. Most women will oblige in giving you a massage before a fuck, but not all with the same professionalism that Carmen does.

Part of the guarantee for getting good service is to choose the right woman. You eventually are able to get a feel for the women just by speaking to them before making any commitment. Many girls are learning to speak English but knowing their language is always a plus. If a girl shows true interest in you then you know you are in for good service, as a lot really do take pleasure in having sex.

A simple test to see if the woman is really enjoying the sex with you is a wet pussy. The way they position their pussy when fucking them can also be a sign. If she positions herself in the way that her clit will rub against your cock or body, then you know she is really into pleasing herself. There is also a way you can tell if she had a real orgasm or was just faking it. They say that when a woman has an orgasm you can sometimes see a physical sign. The area all around her pelvis can become red, almost the same as a blushing face would become red. It is possible though this occurs due to friction.

Patricia was a 19 year old hot Colombian who would close her legs together with your cock deep inside her. She would then be between your legs. That way she would receive maximum contact with her clit. It is quite an accomplishment to make a working girl have a genuine orgasm. Certainly only a few of us can say we made them cum. The highest honor I have ever received after satisfying a hooker was her comment she made to me in Spanish "you are a professional at sex". Truth is that I had such a good chemistry with her that there was genuine sexual passion from my part. My cock and her pussy, fitted like a glove on a hand or how a sword fits into its sheath. When there is a genuine chemistry connection between a couple you are both very likely able to please each other, without fear of been sexually inadequate.

Adriana II would never rush her clients. She preferred to spend quality time with them ensuring they received the service they paid for. If a customer outside was banging on the door hoping to speed up the present customer, she would continue her service at ease. She was into many different fantasies accommodating many men's needs. She was always prepared to go the extra mile just to please her customer.

She loved doggy style so that she could see herself in the mirror being fucked. She was always dressed sexy with high heels. It was a turn on to see her sexy legs parted with a small tattoo on her ankle. She would never take off her high heels while being fucked which added excitement, spicing up the moment.

Maria was a tall elegant sensual black woman from Colombia. At the age of 28 she had worked a number of occasions at Campo. She would start with a full body massage, massaging you all over including your feet. She would end the massage with you lying on your back, while she begins to suck on your nipples. Sucking of the nipples is a very common thing that

Latino girls seem to do to men. She gently sucks on your nipple and sensually caresses your cock and balls. This is a pleasure that results in an extremely hard cock, ready for action. Feeling her pussy you will find it wet as ever. With your cock hard, she then mounts you, and fucks you with mutual pleasure. She moves her body to a pleasurable ritual, her firm brown breasts glistering in the dark. Skillfully she brings you to an explosive orgasm, draining all the cum your balls can offer.

Some time ago I mistakenly offered a hot 19 Colombian girl more money if she gave exceptionally good service. After an average fuck I paid her the going rate of 50 Guilders, which resulted in the old joke of how do you make a "whore moan?" Pay her less money. This whore did moan though, as she claimed she gave me good service, including open mouth kissing. After I refused to pay the excess she locked me in the room and would not let me out. This was a new experience for me and I wasn't sure how to handle it. It was the only time in my life where I was held hostage by a hooker. I wondered to myself at the time about whether I should force my way out? Eventually I paid the 25 Guilder ransom, and was freed by my captive.

Stephanie had her own technique of seducing potential customers. She worked at Stellaris back in the nineties. She was a beautiful sensual Colombian woman about 5' 4" with long silky dark hair. She would sensually rub up against a client in the bar. If they did not show too much interest or who would claim they are not interested in having a woman at that moment. She would invite them up to her room telling them they did not have to pay or did not have to have sex. Once in the room she would lay close up next to the man caressing or massaging him. In no time the man would become aroused, they would surrender to her sexual power and have sex with her. At the end they would feel obligated to pay her for the great service she had supplied. I knew of many men that fell victim to her spell.

A simple test you can do to see if the woman is "just business" is to ask her if she takes the money upfront or after. If she says after, you are almost guaranteed good service. Most women who will take money up front will be the "just business" type and will rush to finish you. I have to note that some women take the money upfront for security reasons, as there have been cases where the men have skipped out without paying. As an honorable customer I think this is bad form when a man does this, as some of these women are fucking to feed their families back home.

CHAPTER 8
RELIGION AND SUPERSTITION

Interesting to note the majority of the working girls are surprisingly religious. Often a Bible is open on a particular page on a table in the same room they perform their sexual services. Latin girls are primarily Catholics. On Good Friday, most of them will not work. They would lock their rooms and only open for business after 12am. I remember Adriana would make a lot of money on this day, as she would be one of the few girls opening her legs for business.

I even came across a woman who had the statue of the Virgin Mary in her room. She would cover it with a cloth when she was servicing her customers. She worked out of a room in a old colonial style building, down a dark alley in Pietermaai, Curacao. She would stand on the corner where the alley met the main road in search of business.

I met another Dominican I call the Lady in Red. She was a married woman, who would wear a sexy red dress and stand on the street by the Catholic Church. I used her services a few times but only for blowjobs.

We would drive to the baseball field, located off a main road and park in back. I would pull down my pants while she would kneel on the passenger seat. She would brush her long brown hair back, and then do the "sign of the cross" before going down on me. Probably she would pray silently "forgive me Father for what I am about to receive". It made me feel sacrilegious and important at the same time. She would suck me off without a condom and knew at the right time to pull her head away, so that she does not get cum in her mouth. She was very pretty woman with a beautiful face. One time I shot my load so much that when she pulled her head away, I shot right over my shoulder. She remarked "mucha leche" (plenty of milk). Luckily, my head was slightly to the left, or I would have cum on my own face.

There are many superstitions some the girls believe and try in order to bring more money. They place cloves in an apple and put it on the dressing table or hang an aloe plant over their door. There is also special lucky or holy water they sell to wash the room with, also to bring luck or money.

I am normally not a superstitious person, but I believe I have witnessed its unusual power. I owned a large house where I rented rooms out daily, weekly or sometimes for just 4 hours. I went through a time when business was a bit slow. Business was good for the 4 hour rate, as we would supply condoms in the rooms. I even had some prominent men from Curacao who used my place to take the girlfriends they had on the side. One man, head of a certain government department would rent the room for a day. One by one he would bring different woman to fuck there, as many as 3-4 in the day.

I mentioned to my Dominican wife who managed the rooms for me, that business was very slow. She said she will take care of it. A few days later I saw cars parked and business booming again. When I asked what she did, she said I would laugh at her and tell her she is crazy. Then she informed me that she had used this "special" water. The Colombian maid we had cleaned the tiled floors in all the rooms with the special water. I replied "Hey if it works, why not!" Was it the water or just coincidence? Who knows, but business had picked up.

I do not look at prostitution as a sin or think badly of the customers that frequent them. I see it as charity as most of the women are working to feed or help their poor families. Of which I am doing my charitable duty to help the poor. Even Jesus befriended a whore, Mary Magdalene. If he can be a friend of a whore then so can we. I should be knighted for all my charitable work over the years.

For many of these women it is not a question of sin, but a question of survival. Most of these women are devoted Christians, who will attend church regularly. Even in Amsterdam there is a church in the Red Light district surrounded by the famous window prostitutes.

A Foreign executive manager living in the Islands came out with a brilliant plan. He inquired how much a teacher earns in Colombia, which was about $200 a month. So he offered a position of a combination maid and mistress for the same amount of money. Strange as it might seem, it turned out to be a priest who found him such a woman from Colombia. A beautiful young woman with long dark hair took the position. They ended up falling in love and eventually married. However, they did not live happily ever after. She traded him in for an airline pilot some years later. He ended up losing his mind and living on the streets. He was later found dead in an abandoned building. It is amazing how a person can go from a position of statue to a bum on the street. I saw him just a week before he died looking for food in a garbage container. I gave him 10 guilders and told him to get something to eat. He spoke as if his mind was all there at the time. As they say some lose all will to live a normal life.

A high class hooker named Maria from Santiago Chile donated 27 hours of her time for charity. She charged $300 per hour for sexual encounters with her and managed to collect a total of $5400. That works out to be about 18 customers in the 27 hours. On her website she posted a copy of the bank deposit slip as proof that the money went to the charity. Wish we had more women like that.

One would ask if there is a Patron Saint for hookers. Well there is one, Saint Nicholas. Hookers have always looked up to him after he helped three hookers with some coins.

CHAPTER 9
FEMALE CLIENTS

I had a lesbian friend who would regularly visit the hot spots in pursuit of female company. She would chat them up as any other regular guy and take them back to her place or to their hotel rooms. She was one of the very few or possibly the only female customer that was allowed into Campo back then, likely because of her butch looks.

Now as times have changed, women are demanding equal opportunity. Campo now allows women to visit on Tuesdays but they have to pay a higher entrance fee than the men. You can always tell the visiting women from the working women by the simple fact they are carrying handbags. You will never see a working girl from Campo carrying a handbag during working hours. The Russian woman who worked at Campo was the only one I ever saw who would have a handbag with her.

One Tuesday we decided to visit to see how these nights were going. I noticed one of the rooms being frequented by many of the women clientele. There were even two women entering at a time. I wondered who this woman in the room was. She must be an expert in pleasing all these women, as they all came out the room looking very much relieved. Turned out they were using the room for the toilet. Previously there was never any need for female public toilets. The working women would use their own toilets in their rooms.

A nightclub previously known as the "Rode Lion" (Red Lion) had female clients. They would enjoy the nightly exotic shows and indulge in their own obsession of having a female whore. I asked one of the girls working there if she would service these customers. She eagerly replied yes and said many of the girls obliged these services. She remarked it was a pleasure to be paid for someone to caress and satisfy them for a change.

In some of the other locations like LTs, it was common to see European and local couples in search of lovely Latin girls for a threesome. They would both enjoy watching the girls dancing. Select a beautiful young Latin woman, and then leave with her for a night of steamy sexual pleasures.

It has become more acceptable for women to enjoy seeing other women perform the sensual, erotic acts. Even in the United States there are strip joints which cater only to women clientele, with female exotic dancers for their entertainment. In the Nevada whorehouse ranches they have female customers.

CHAPTER 10

FROM THE BOYS

Juan Carlos is one of my friends who I can claim has had the most experience on this subject. His favorite was "fuck them in their ass". He would ask, as his Spanish was not very good, "Ask her if she gives the Kulu?" "Kulu" is the local Papiamentu word for ass. He also had a preference for darker girls. He would make them go on all fours. Grab their ass with both hands and spread the cheeks apart like a ripe fruit, then spit right on her ring piece. Slowly he'd insert his thumb to widen and test the hole before inserting his dick into her ass. He would hear them groan with pain or pleasure as he pushed his way deeper and deeper. After his encounters he'd walk back to the bar wiping the sweat from his brow and say "Ooh that was a good one, she took it in the ass all the way" gesturing with his hand the depth of his penetration.

Some jealous hooker named Danielle was pissed off with Norman for seeing him with another hooker. So one day she went to his work at a hotel to change some money. She got a ride home with him and on the way she confronted him about his indiscretions. She threatened to kill him, eventually attacking him with a knitting needle. This frightened him and is what actually led to his hasty departure from Curacao. The fear of what some deranged Colombian hooker might do, or arrange to have done to him if he ever dared to sleep around again. Believe me he was dead scared. A friend had suggested to him to threaten her with immigration, but he decided it was best to leave whilst in one piece. Some of these women do get a little jealous if you've been seeing one of them and then decide to try out another. They'll give you the "stink" eye or notion with two fingers on the head symbolizing horns.

In the Caribbean Islands if you ever want to make these women disappear, walk into one of these bars where most women are illegal and shout "Immigration!" Next thing you will notice is just how quickly they vacate the premises.

Chris finished off his nightshift and decided to go up the road to Campo. Still in his suit, he met a woman named Losdairio from Room 99. She was known for giving excellent blowjobs. Chris decided to have one, but he did not know at the time that she had a problem with her jaw. A few minutes into the blowjob he heard her complaining, lifting up her head lips apart. She had succumbed to lock jaw. Soon the Watchyman turned up when they had thought Chris had hit the girl. It was quickly realized what had happened. Chris felt sorry for the girl, feeling partially responsible due to the size of his dick. He rushed her to the hospital still dressed in his suit. Hooker at his arm and mouth jammed open. Must have been awkward moment explaining to the Doctors what had happened. He ended up leaving the hospital at midday the next morning. His boss at that time remarked to him when he showed up for work the next evening, "It's your big dick that landed you in this". Needless to say by this time the story had spread around the Island like wild fire.

Jim found a woman at the Camp who had a different look to her. A few days before a friend had told him about a sex change hooker working at LTs. As he was fucking away the thought of the sex change had crossed his mind. He stopped in mid-stride, pulled his dick out of her and was curious if she was not a sex change. Parting her legs, he examined her pussy only to find she had a natural pussy with a clit. The woman asked what he was doing. He casually remarked he just wanted to see her pussy before he shot his load.

A few years ago, I had a friend who mentioned he had been with a sex change. The reason he knew was that he could not stick his dick all the way because her pussy had not been too deep. Another of the other telltale signs is if the woman has an Adams' apple.

Al had found a 32 year old Colombian at La Tasca and accompanied her to her room at Hotel Carlos across the street. She was a pretty, dark haired woman very new to the business. Unlike most women starting in the late teens or early twenties, she only got into the business at 32. As he was lying on his back with her on top he finally joyously shot his load. He lay there on the bed catching his breath as she dismounted. He then heard her saying in Spanish "Oh my God, Oh my God", wiping her forehead staring at his dick. Hearing this he thought wow he was really that good, thinking that she was saying this out of pleasurable exhaustion. Then he noticed that the condom had broken, being some cheap unknown brand. He's often wondered if one of his swimmers had reached one of her eggs. Personally I've often wondered how many pregnancies have resulted in these kinds of mishaps to working girls.

Punta Cana, Dominican Republic was the setting for Tony's story. He was in a bar that had about 20 working girls. There was a mixture of all types of women. A tall woman with long hair eyed him, smiling at him. Slowly she worked her way to Tony greeting him with a smile as she was moving her body to the music. Something about the woman's look had him curiously wondering if it was a transvestite or shemale.

So he decided to do a test. In his broken Spanish he asked if he could touch her below, which she obliged. He stroked his hand between her legs, her jeans tightly fitted against her thighs. There seemed to be no sign of a penis. Although still weary, his curiosity got the better of him and invited her back to the hotel room. Back in the room he removed his pants. She immediately moved like lightening to her knees, grabbing his dick and started sucking desperately. He sat down on the bed as she carried on sucking him vigorously. He made her pause and asked her to take her jeans off. She hesitated and asked him if he was sure about it. Low and behold as the jeans came down and the panties pulled down to her knees, a large cock appeared. Satisfied that he had quelled his curiosity, he let "her/him" finish giving him the blow job, shooting his cum in "her/his" mouth. Moral of the story: Beware some transvestites are good at hiding their dicks and balls.

Juan Carlos claims to have fucked about 2000 hookers over the years. We sat down and did the math, which turned out to be plausible. Speaking of breaking records! He did break my bed in the spare room, fucking a Dominican woman.

A girlfriend once asked me how many hookers I had met. At the time I gave her a conservative estimate of 600. After more thought and consideration my count of over 20 years' history is more likely in the region of over 1000 women.

Chris told Juan Carlos one day about how cheap he was. He said "You only gave her an extra 10 guilder compensation?! "This was after a willing girl at Campo gave him her ass for the first time. It was a tight one for Juan Carlos. He had to force his 9" dick slowly into her tight hole. After he shot his load she ran to the bathroom to wipe her ass. To her horror she discovered blood. That is when Juan Carlos grinned at her and pulled out the extra 10 to compensate her for the pain and blood.

This story from Juan Carlos involves a mixture of alcohol, Viagra, rush and probably a bit of weed. He was so horny one night after work that he had to go up to Campo for a fuck. Walking around he observed all the women who were available that night until he stopped at room 131. A slightly older woman with dark hair had captured his attention and with the Viagra starting to kick in he entered the room, his cock now protruding straight out. Fortunately she was able to speak some English as his request was just to get a blowjob. She began sucking his hard cock as he sniffed at the rush, amplifying the sensation. He then pulled out his cock and asked her to lie on her back head over the end of the bed. With one hand over her throat he began to throat fuck her, pushing his cock all the way deep down her throat. He fucked away feeling like a porn star, noticing she was enjoying this. He finally shot his load. The woman stood up rubbing her throat and said "well that is enough throat fucking for the night." The next night he returned to look for her as this was the best throat fuck he had ever had. She was occupied, so he ended up in room 167with a 25 year old slim Colombian replacement. For an extra 25 guilders she was willing to give him her ass. Once again loaded with alcohol, Viagra and the rush bottle in hand, he fucked her hard up the ass. The more abuse he gave her, the more she seemed to enjoy it as he could feel that her pussy was so wet. After a while she started complaining as her ass was starting to get sore. Realizing her pain he pulled his cock out and made her kneel down to finish him off with a blowjob. For an extra 25 guilders she was willing to take a cum shot without a condom. Once again he felt like a porn star as he shot his cum into her mouth and all over her face. After this the woman remarked "you are my man". With the extras the 100 guilder experience was well worth it.

Jim had met Carmen the 19 year old Dominican at a Strip club called "The Tunnel". This was a place situated on one of the back streets between Holiday Beach and the Marriott hotels. The building consisted of two levels, two bars downstairs with the dance floor and another smaller cozy bar upstairs. From the upper level you could look down onto the dance floor. What made this place interesting was that they would only have young dancers between the ages of 18 and 24, mostly from Dominican Republic. It was also the only place I know of in Curacao where you could get a hand job while sitting at the bar. Carmen was working behind the bar on the upper level when Jim had met her. He was so turned on by her that he knew he had to have her, so he asked her if he could have sex with her. She said "yes" but told him only when she finished her shift. It just shows you what a man will go through just to get the pussy he really wanted. He sat at the bar for over six hours waiting for her to finish her shift. Jim went through a period of been drunk to sobering up just waiting for her. At about 3am he could not wait any longer, so he asked Carmen to see if her Manager would let her take some time off. Fortunately the Manager agreed, so they rushed to the apartment she was staying at next to the building. When they reached her apartment, they both realized they did not have a condom. Carmen quickly rushed to the other women's apartments in search of a condom, but to no avail. So Jim who was so horny at this time settled for the best thing. No, it was not a hand job or blowjob. He had what some would call "play sex", placing his cock in between her legs close to her sweet pussy, her smooth thighs stroking his cock until he shot his load on her sheets.

Andrew mentioned to me he will never go into room 126 no matter how hot the woman is. As two men have actually died in the room. One of apparently died from a heart attack from a snorting too much coke and the other of a heart attack caused by Viagra. Both men probably died smiling.

The following story is from a Dutch friend Eddy in his own words.

"Here the stories I promised you. You can experience some adventure in this Sodom and Gomorra. Last week I was with 2 friends in a bar where I met a sexy Colombian chick. I thought this is or a hooker or a Colombian girl who wants to get fucked by a Dutch guy. Because I believe in the good of people I assumed the latter.

After we talked for a while (she Spanish and I Papiamentu), did she say that she wanted to go home with me. Because she looked very sexy I said let's go. When we came to my house she came right to business. She was a hooker! And not a cheap one! She wanted Naf. 450,—for the whole night. The value for money was nowhere to be found because she was not that hot. While I was thinking if I should pay the money, she had started doing coke. Because I was drunk and horny I agreed, but I had only Naf. 150,—and told her that she would get the rest the next morning.

We were on the bed and she kept on doing coke and wining about the rest of the money. She gave me some coke, the first time in my life. First I thought that it did nothing to me but later I think it did. I started to get pretty irritated because she kept on wining about the money and all of a sudden I had enough of her. I told her to shut up and put on her clothes because I was going to bring her back to the bar. She was very surprised but probably because of the way I said it she felt there was no room for discussion. She put on her clothes and we went back to the bar. I'm telling you, the whole damn 45 minutes drive we have been fighting. She kept on asking and screaming what was wrong and I was being grumpy. All of a sudden It was like I watched the whole situation through the eyes of a third person and I saw a Colombian coke hooker arguing with a Dutch country boy and I had to laugh very hard inside myself and had trouble staying in my role. When we came to the bar I kicked her out and drove home.

The next morning I woke up sober and thanked God that she was not next to me and that nothing happened.

After a break up with an Antillean woman I had a crush on. I decided closed the book regarding her, but was still very frustrated about the whole situation, so I decided to go to Campo Alegre, a place with about 150 sexy Colombian and Dominican prostitutes. You should see it, all the girls are so sexy, you don't know where to look. Anyway, after all that shit with my ex I thought I had deserved a trip to this place to forget about it. First I went to the Casino and when you're not lucky in love than in the Casino. I won $ 1.000,—and with my pockets full with money I went to Campo. My plan was to fuck more than one woman that night because I had never done that before. And because of all the booze I already drank the reformed education of my parents had already drowned in the alcohol and was not in my way.

I was together with a friend, who I lost within 5 minutes and then met another friend. He recommended me a certain lady, but because she was not black I told him I was not interested. You ever heard 'If you go black, you'll never go back'? Well, that's true. While I told him I was looking for a black girl, I saw a pretty black girl passing by and winking me. She was almost 6 feet, had long hair, a sweet face and a nice body. She was going to be #1 this evening! Imagine Campo as a crossing between the 'Wallen' in Amsterdam and a holiday camp. You have 150 little houses in which the girls stay for 3 months till their working permit expires. We went to her little house and I was very excited. And she too! While I was still taking of my pants she already started sucking my cock without a condom. And how! My cock has been sucked before in the past but never like this! This was something else. She was a suck artist. And with the fucking (I will keep the details for myself) she went straight to the # 1 position on my list of best fucks. I have been to hookers in Holland and that was ok, but not like this, this was fantastic.

But of course I had to stick to the plan to fuck 5 girls that night, so when I almost came I jumped of the bed and told her I had to leave. She looked at me with a face of complete disbelieve and asked me if I had come. She looked so sad I felt sorry for her. She walked with me to the bar and there I told her I had to look for my friend. So I went to find #2 for that evening. I saw a blond Colombian girl with a beautiful face and body. She spoke English (most of them don't) and seemed very nice. She told me if I would go with her it would be spectacular and I was very curious *for that. But unfortunately. He was boring. While fucking her I regret leaving #1. So I told this girl too I had to leave and this one got angry. I told her I drank too much and I would come back another time. I went to check for my friend and who do I meet? Yes, #1 again. She asked me if I already had found my friend and I told her no. Then she asked me if I wanted to come with her again and I said of course! It was even better than the first time. But I had drunk so much that I could not come anymore. In order to make she come she sucked my cock while she jerked me off so hard that my dick hurt for 4 days.*

The days after this night I sat on my work with a hard dick all the time. Every time I was thinking about #1 it got hard again. One thing was for sure, when my dick would not hurt anymore, I would go back to her. So, after 5 days I went back and the first girl I see was #2, but I ignored her. Later she saw me with #1 and after that she ignored me. Well, this time was even better than the first 2. She told me she loved me and wanted to be my girlfriend. After this time I went again and again and again and every time was better than the time before that. Unfortunately she is back in Cali, Colombia because she had to go back, so I have to wait 5 months for her to come back."

CHAPTER 11

FROM THE GIRLS

Erika was the Russian woman who spent a few months at Campo training the girls how to dance. She was tall, tattooed, short dark hair and spoke English fluently. She enjoyed the work, both dancing and fucking for money. She was aware of the low going rate of 50 guilders at the Camp, as she was normally used to the higher rates. What pissed her off were guys who would approach her for a quick fuck and offer her 25 guilders. She preferred to spend quality time with each customer slowly working up to heavy erotic passion. She accepted the going rate but would gladly appreciate if the customer gave her more. Many did as she gave excellent service.

It was a known fact that most of the young locals would offer the girls 25 guilders for a quick one, as they did not have much money. Many girls would oblige if business was slow. One could get the bargain price in the early hours after midnight, when the girls were about to retire for the night. A quick 25 guilders at the end of the night would pay for their meals the next day.

A while back I met up with Diana, a tall Dominican in her early thirties, who managed to maintain her body in slim healthy condition. She was a fun girl always up for private parties involving lesbian shows. Diana said that she was staying in a stylish two-bedroom apartment. I asked her if she had a rich boyfriend who was paying for the apartment. She responded by tapping her pussy and saying "this is what pays for the apartment". She shared the apartment with her younger sister of 24 who had a very similar body but tighter pussy. The sisters were up to threesomes but would only get more intimate with each other in a show where they could make more money.

One of Andréa's best days for working at the Camp was on Good Friday. As mentioned before most girls do not work on this day because of religious reasons. She was not so religious herself and would be open to business. On this day she would make very good money as the men would be willing to pay higher prices for her time due to limited choices. She was a prime selection. She did not charge a higher price that day, but I think they felt obliged to give her extra due to the great service she gave.

Recently I met up with Ella, a tall sexy Colombian who I had been with years ago. I decided to give her a second chance and try her out again. I was more attracted to her this time as she had changed her hair back to her natural color, which was black. For years she had plied her business as a blonde. She noted to me that it has been 10 years that she has been in the business. It was obvious she had with some surgical enhancements that included a tummy tuck and breast implants. She surprised me stating she remembered me as I was her first customer. She had started at Campo back in 1998. Over the 10 years she had worked 7 times at Campo. Her resume would reflect other locations in the Caribbean such as Saint Marten, Panama and Aruba.

Ella started her career in the sex business back in Colombia in 1998. The father of her child would not support her or the child. She had to fend for herself. The easiest option was to go into prostitution. She started out at a discrete house called "Casa Reservado", run by an old woman. Usually young women working there. The going rate at this house was 30,000 pesos, about $15 for a quickie. Her first client was a thirty year old man who treated her like badly, but she had to tolerate this as she desperately needed the money to survive. At first she did not enjoy the sex at all. Later she learned to enjoy it as she met plenty of men with good hearts and who treated her well. After a few weeks of work she made enough money to buy her mother a color TV, which was a privileged item to own back then. She was so proud of the fact that she had earned to money to buy her mother such a gift. This is where she learnt about the opportunity to work in Curacao, Aruba and St Marten. Ella once mentioned to me that if we continued our friendship outside of the walls of Campo, I must never ask her or remind her about her work as a puta.

Linda was a European woman who only started her career in prostitution in her forties. She told me that she was lucky at her first encounter. She was nervous about doing it the first time. Her first client turned out to be a good looking young Dutchman with an average size cock. So this made her first time a bit easy as she was attracted to him. She was worried about how she would feel after this. Would she feel guilty or dirty? Instead she was thrilled remarking "bring on my next client". She soon realized of course that not all the clients would be appealing, and had to learn to switch off her mind and fuck for the money.

One night I was standing at the bar drinking with Juan Carlos, when Julie joined us for a drink. She spoke perfect English and soon joined into the conversation that Juan Carlos and I were having. I was mentioning the fact that you know when you have a true connection to a hooker's heart. This is when she tells you her real name. Immediately Julie blurted out her real name. I was taken aback by this sudden revelation from her. We continued to have an intelligent conversation with her about the sex business. She claims that 60% of the women in the business are in it purely for the financial gain. The other 40% just enjoy the sex, drugs and partying. Her first time was with a business man from Puerto Rico who was visiting Colombia on business. He offered her $500 for sex, which opened her eyes to a whole new world of money and sex. Her father drank a lot and was not able to support their family. Her new found venture, and five years on, was able to help pay for both her and sister through college.

This one probably belongs to "Ripley's believe it or not". In 2010 I came across Katy, a 22 year old Colombian woman working out of room 120 at Campo. When I passed by we greeted one another. Her beauty caught my attention. She was about 5'2" dark hair and a naughty look about her. I passed her by though and went around the corner. Thinking about it there was something about her that sparked my interest in her, so I turned around to go back to her. In those few short moments she was already surrounded by four guys. There must have been some connection between us as she looked over and noticed me. She then slowly walked away from the four guys to meet up with me.

It was her first time at Campo. One month into her three month stay, and 15 months into her new career.

She had started her career as a hooker in Panama at a club with a going rate of $25 for a 15 minute quickie. This surprised me as I always thought that Campo's $28 rate was the lowest in the area. She claims to have serviced 42 men in one day while working at the club in Panama. Rubbing her stomach she explained to me her body had been in pain after taking on so many men. This surprised me as it even beat Lisa's record of 18 men in one night.

I asked her how many men had she had that very night we met, to which she explained to me she had been with 8 men. I asked her if this was true. She immediately led me to her bathroom, reached into her small garbage can situated next to the toilet. Scratching around she removed some paper towels to reveal the used condoms. With a quick glance I could count 5 condoms, so it is very possible that 3 lay somewhere beneath the paper towels. It was only 11pm on a Friday night, so she must have had many more after that.

I had to test drive her. I had to give her a 10/10 for beauty, body, service and attitude. She had no children, natural small breasts, small waistline, a small tattoo on her left upper thigh, ankle chain on her right leg. I have a thing about ankle chains. I think they are so sexy, especially when you see it on a sexy leg as you fuck away. She was very open to fantasies, and allowing men to cum on her back, tits or face. She explained that when she sees men excited, that in return excites her. Another surprising thing about her was that she revealed to me her fantasy. At first I had mistaken it for that she wanted anal, which I quickly told her I had a friend Juan Carlos that would love to try her. I soon learnt that it was that she wanted to give a man anal using a strap on dildo. She was standing at the edge of the bed gesturing how she would fuck the guy up the ass. She gave me her personal phone number as I was curious to know if she would have fulfilled her fantasy before leaving Campo. *Answer to follow*

CHAPTER 12
DON'T JUDGE A BOOK BY ITS COVER

As I might have mentioned before, one of our code words for Campo was "The Library", so wives or girlfriends would not know what we are talking about. So this is about some of the "books" we came across.

While walking around at Campo I came across a girl with a good body but shame about her face. I walked up to her and started speaking to her. While we were talking she was looking around. This is normally a sign that she is just business, as she was looking around for the next customer incase I rejected her. Instead she was not focusing her attention on me. So I walked away knowing that it would be just business and a rushed service.

Later that night I decided to give her advice on the matter. I explained to her that she should make eye contact with a potential customer and not look around while they are talking to her. She agreed with my observation and told me I am right, as she was studying marketing. One of the points she was taught during a business marketing lesson was to make eye contact with the customer.

She told me she gives a great massage. So I decided to give her a chance. Turned out to be one of the best services I have had in a while. She gave me an unrushed full body massage, including a foot massage, followed by an intense fuck.

So the lesson I had learned was don't judge a book by its cover. Normally you can use good judgment as mentioned in Chapter 7, Good Service. Sometimes there are those who just need a little help in selling their product.

A friend of mine had remarked that he had a friend who would only fuck large woman. They would give the best fuck as they would not know when their next one would be. Funny enough, when out with a bunch of guys he would generally be the one that would always got laid.

Over the years I have met plenty of women in this line of business who have beautiful sexy bodies, but not such pretty faces. I have to say most of them were known for their great service. To find a fully beautiful girl from top to bottom that can give good service is obviously a bonus.

Some time ago I came across a beautiful dark haired, 5' 5" Colombian woman full of tattoos on her legs and arms. My first impression was that she looked like a wild biker type chick. However, after speaking to her for awhile I realized she was actually quite a sweet pleasant woman. She gave a gentle, sensual, erotic service.

A plumpish not so good looking Colombian woman who would not get much visual notice turned out to be a top earning hooker at Campo. Apparently she would give great service catering to all kinds of fetishes. In a three month period at Campo, she had made over $22,000. One of her clients would pay her 600 guilder ($333) confidentially to stick a dildo up his ass.

CHAPTER 13
QUALITY CONTROL

If there was ever a job I could choose and know I would be good at, it would be a Quality Control Officer in a whorehouse. This is a job I would be a professional at and take great pleasure doing.

When I look around a whorehouse like Campo, I look at the girls and am able to access and examine them. From what they are wearing to how they walk or present themselves. Some of the working girls tend to under estimate the importance on how they present themselves. A mature Ukrainian woman I know who had worked in the fashion business in Europe once told me how import it is "how" a woman in the sex business dresses. If she dresses classy, she will tend to fetch a higher price for her sexual services. Trashy will not get you top dollar.

This is a business where first impressions do count. Sexy high heel shoes are always a turn on. Mind you there are some women who either don't know how to walk in them or it just does not suit their walk. These girls should stay in their rooms showing off their sexy legs in high heels, instead of prancing around like "an elephant with horseshoes" A comment a friend of mine made while we were both observing a tall sexy woman prancing around Campo, was how her clumsy walk did not do her any justice. A woman does not have to have extreme high heels, even a 3" heel can do the job.

Flat shoes are generally a turn off in this line of business, but there are some men who do find this attractive. Flat shoes can go well with certain sexy attire. A barefoot beauty with painted toenails can be extremely sexy with the right type of girl. Painted toenails always add to a sexy look. One should try fucking a woman with her high heeled shoes still on with sexy painted toenails. At Campo they have large mirrors next to the beds. You can see her sexy feet in the high heels as you penetrate her deeply.

The sight of a schoolgirl skirt pulled up to the waist, legs apart, sexy painted toenails slipped into high heels can stimulate the extra blood to flow to your cock, giving you an incredibly good hard on. A schoolgirl skirt combined with white knee or thigh high stockings is also a great sexy look. Occasionally at Campo you will find such women.

I had a hot 19 year old Colombian in high heels, standing on one leg, bent over, the other leg resting on top of the cabinet. While I fucked her from behind, I could see even she was enjoying this. She was watching herself in the mirror enjoying the feeling of a hard stiff cock penetrating her. This position and her sexy look added to the pleasure.

How they dress can have first impressions for some, but I have to say that there are men who don't get turned on by what the women are wearing. They must have other standards or quality control requirements. Different strokes for different folks, I suppose.

Lately more and more girls at Campo have been wearing flat shoes. If I had my way I would send them back to the room to change. Wearing flat shoes to go have their meals at the cafeteria are ok for me. On the "job", it should be heels.

A friend would tell me, don't fuck them just after they have eaten. Her full stomach might slow down her erotic moves. So try and avoid visiting them during meal times, or make sure you fuck them before they eat.

There is an unfortunate quality that most experienced men would notice. It is orange peel skin or also referred to as "hail damage". With the older working girls cellulite sets in. The firmness gives way to loose wobbly jelly like asses and hips. Most women either don't notice this or don't care, but it is noticed by the keen eye of some clients. If a man had a young whore with a tight body, they would normally state that her body was so firm that you could bounce a quarter off her.

CHAPTER 14

AROUND THE WORLD

Some of the countries where Prostitution is legal are places like Canada, Britain, Australia and New Zealand. Surprisingly in Holland it was not legal at first, but like most countries prostitution is normally tolerated and not criminally enforced. Since then prostitution has become legal.

One of the most interesting places for the sex business in the world has to be Amsterdam. The main red light district is situated on the east side of Damrak near the Central Station. Window shopping is the key to finding the girls, as most of the girls work in small rooms that either have a glass door or window, so they can display their goods to potential customers. You could walk the cobbled streets and look up to see all the women in the windows. Some windows are situated in a building. So it's like walking around a small shopping mall, window shopping for a sexual treat. There are even windows right next to a church, located in the infamous red light district.

The Red Light district name comes from the early days before electricity. A street prostitute would walk around with a red burning lantern. This was used to hold up to their face, so that a potential customer could see what she looks like. Even nowadays you can spot the odd red light placed at an apartment window at night indicating there is a woman open for business.

Some years back when Holland still had the Dutch Guilder the going rate was 50 guilders for about half an hour. Now they have the Euro it is still "50". It seems to have been the standard with the Dutch. With Curacao being a Dutch Island, the Campo rate is still 50 guilders to this day.

There seems to be certain areas of the red light district where the same culture or nationalities seem to gather. You will find streets with mostly Dutch girls. Other locations have mostly black, Latina or Oriental girls. There was a street I found that had all beautiful Thai women. Warning though if you do venture down Bloedstraat, this is where you will find the transvestites and shemales. I did take a walk once down there out of curiosity. I have to say one or two of them looked pretty much like real women. The ones in bikini panties seemed to hide their cocks so well. Some of them did look obviously like transvestites as some were quite tall or had masculine features still present. I came across a petite one from Venezuela right at the end of the lane. I was convinced that she must be a natural female. I was able to speak to her in Spanish asking her if she was female or shemale. She finally convinced me that she was a shemale by lifting up her skirt, pulled her panties to the side to reveal a small dick. If you did not know this, you would be convinced that she was a real woman. Just makes you think, how many hot sexy women that you might have seen could actually have been a transsexual?

Recently the Authorities have tried to make their work more legitimate, by getting the girls to pay taxes. This surprisingly attracted more local Dutch girls to the business, to fill in the vacancies left by illegal immigrants fearing getting caught. Some of the young Dutch girls even had support from their parents. They would say at least their daughter was out working, instead of them unemployed hanging around the house.

In a TV interview a Dutch woman stated her case as to why she was in the business. She would have to work eight hours in a bar just to make 50 Euro and still have to pay the baby sitter for looking after her kid while she was at work. With her working just one shift in one of the windows she could easily make about 300 Euro for the night.

Many countries try to combat street prostitution. In Amsterdam they had a special zoned area for street prostitutes to do their business. In 1996 the zoned area at Theemsweg was referred to as the Municipal Brothel. They even had car cubicles you could drive into, to give you some privacy to do your business. Unfortunately this place was closed down in 2003.

It has never been illegal to exchange sex for money in Canada, but there are many laws against the surrounding activities. Prostitution is legal as long as the soliciting is done behind closed doors. It is illegal to solicit sex in public and only one prostitute can work under one location. This law prevents brothels from springing up. Most girls will advertise themselves as escorts or masseuses.

Massage parlors are in any Canadian city or town. In Niagara Falls they are mostly located in Lundy's Lane near the Strip places. There is normally a room fee of about $30 to $40, and then you tip the woman for extras which could range from $40 for a hand job to $100 or more for sex. I have come across a place where a mature Eastern European woman would only charge $20 extra for what she calls a "hand release". She had a wonderful sensual way of doing it, caressing very lightly. It was so good my cum shot as far as my shoulder, in several squirting intervals. The woman even remarked how much I had cum. This was probably the best value hand job I have ever received in my life.

A comment I have heard and experienced for myself about the Canadian women is that they do not have an attitude like their Southern neighbors. Along with the normally weaker Canadian Dollar, many men from the USA venture across the border for good value and a good time with the Canadian women.

I was surprised when I had my first lap dance in Canada. I sat with my arms straight by my sides, afraid I would have a bouncer pounce on me if I touched her, like they would do in the USA. The sexy French Canadian woman politely told me that I was allowed to touch her. Allowing me to touch her nice firm breasts and run my hands up and down her smooth body.

A female friend once accompanied me to the same place as she also had interest seeing women strip. We met up with the same French Canadian woman. She told us she was into lap dances for couples. She did her lap dance over my wife, making her touch her breasts in the process. Later my wife admitted to me how the experience had turned her on. I always feel I was one of the fortunate ones whose wife was open enough to accompany me or permit me to explore these erotic experiences. I would always tell her that this was research for the book. I am grateful that she was part of my life.

At one of the strip clubs in Lundy's Lane I noticed a job that I never knew existed. There was a well built guy standing next to the stage, who I thought was just a bouncer. When the girls had finished their dance session he would get up on the stage and wipe down the pole, getting it ready for the next dancer. I wondered what he tells his family and friends about the job he does. "I am a pole cleaner, wiping off pussy juice and sweat". This is obviously a requirement for hygienic reasons as I noticed this procedure at Private Eyes in St Catharines. The next dancer would wipe down the pole and railings before they started dancing.

I have noticed that Canadian hookers have a longer career span. The women range from ages 18 all the way up to 64 working in the sex business. I have come across a large number of women in their forties working. I don't know if they had a late start to their career or if they have been working since their 20's. I also noticed a trend in women that do start their career later in life. Most of these women are divorced and this is the best career option that they have. Remember a woman is in her sexual prime in her 40's, unlike a man whose sexual prime is about 20-27 years old.

Some of the women who work in the massage parlors will not go for sex or as they will call it "full service". They will give you great hand jobs with massage oil. This would involve rubbing your balls and cock, sticking their finger up your ass to give you a prostate massage. Some of these women will let you play with their tits, while they massage your dick. Normally the room fee is $40 and anything extra you pay the woman or as they will call it a "tip". A hand job would normally cost you $40 extra.

A Canadian sex-worker from Vancouver claimed that in her 21 year career, starting from the age of 19, that she had over 30,000 clients. In a month she could easily service 500 men.

One thing I always remember about London, England was the telephone booths back in the 80s. I don't know if this is the case now as I have not visited London in a while. If you wanted to find a hooker just go into any telephone booth. They would be filled with stickers of girls advertising themselves. Normally it would be girls who would have their locations nearby, some even walking distance from the booth. There are visible signs from where old stickers had been peeled off. I wondered if that was from the authorities, a Customer keeping the sticker for future use or perhaps the girls themselves removing the competitions stickers.

I did try one of these back in 1985. I had a nice blond English girl for just 40 pounds. Now I hear the price is a lot higher. She was a very pleasant lass who gave great service for the money. Back then street hookers could be found in Soho, which has now been cleaned up quite a bit. Soho was known for its peep shows, sex shops and girls in rooms. The working girls who had apartments or rooms in the area would either have a notice on the front door or at night have a red light in the window. They referred to themselves as "models" on the notices or telephone booth stickers. A typical sign on the door would read "busty blond model available" I was warned that some of the Soho street hookers would run off with the clients' money without giving any service.

The girls who operated out of a room or flat (apartment) normally had another woman around, probably for security reasons. Those who were alone would pretend there was another person present. When they took the money from the client upfront they would disappear for a moment saying they have to give the madam the money. This was a wise ploy they adopted to try and avoid dangerous situations from arising.

Nowadays with the internet most girls advertise themselves through escort sites etc. I did read recently that a lot of college girls in the UK where getting in the business to help pay for their books and tuition. Apparently the authorities were not too happy about this new trend. They can't blame the girl for the choice considering she can make the same money fucking for one hour than working two eight hour shifts as a waitress.

I was surprised to see beautiful street hookers back in 1985 in Tel Aviv, Israel. You would find these stunning women standing on the street for a going rate of $50 at the time. Many of them had long wavy hair, well tanned and fit slim bodies. Even the Israeli female soldiers looked hot with their camouflage pants, t-shirts, and wavy shoulder length hair. I was supposed to get a job as a deckhand/DJ with a pirate radio station called "Voice of Peace", which would broadcast from the middle of the Mediterranean Sea. They only paid you $150 a month. Three weeks at sea and one week in a hotel. Even with these low wages some DJs would start off with this radio station to make a name for themselves. My budget back then was to spend $50 on a hooker during my shore leave, $50 for partying and to save $50 a month. I ended up not taking the job as it was Christmas Eve and missed the Christmas atmosphere there. So I jumped on a plane and flew back to London. Now in Israel they have had an influx of Russian women.

In Greece prostitution is legal. A working girl has to get a personal permit to work as a prostitute. They have to work on the street and not in brothels. In January 2010 prostitutes demonstrated in central Athens to demand licenses to work in brothels. The women wore scarves to hide their identities. They do have brothels in Greece but this is illegal and the women are subject to arrest if caught working in one.

Travel all the way down under and you find a country where prostitution is fully legal. In 2003 New Zealand decriminalized prostitution. Brothels, street prostitution and even pimping is legal. There was a case where a female police officer had a second job working as a prostitute. When the authorities in the city of Auckland found out they told her that although she can take a second job, she cannot work as a prostitute. They said it was because of possible criminal association with the business. She apparently started working part-time as a prostitute because of financial difficulties.

In Auckland, New Zealand a principal found himself in as dilemma when it was reported to him that one of his female teachers, a mother of two in her 30's, was moonlighting as a prostitute. With the stigma attached to prostitution even though it is totally legal and a classed as a legitimate job, he was worried about what the students' parents would think. She was apparently a well liked and good teacher. She defended her position to the principal, stating that her night time work did not interfere with her teaching. The teacher's council said there was no evidence that this had a negative impact on her profession. The Prostitutes Collective national co-coordinator stated there are several teachers who work as prostitutes on the side.

A part-time substitute teacher in the US decided to enter the business as she was not making enough to get by on. She would moonlight as a high class call-girl earning $200 a time. When arrested the police did not use discretion, and just stormed into her room. She was sitting naked on the bed. I think the reason the police officers did it that way was out of curiosity. She was fired from her teaching job, but said that she most regretted the fact that she could not take care of her regular clients. At the time of arrest she commented, "These men needed me. I will miss servicing them" It is not uncommon to find women from all sorts of other professions doing this to make ends meet. One was even a professor at a University, but she committed suicide after she was charged with prostitution. She could not face the shame of been caught.

An Ohio 4th grade school teacher was arrested for prostitution in 2009 after she skipped school to meet up with a client. She had posted an ad on Craigslist. The client that responded was an undercover cop who arrested her in the parking lot of the hotel. The blonde haired teacher had left school claiming she was ill so that she could meet up with the client. She was charged with misdemeanor prostitution and was put on administration leave from the school. She had worked for 13 years as a teacher without any problems. Not sure how many years she had the side job as a prostitute.

In a TV interview a US truck stop hooker remarked that when she stopped hooking it was such a pleasure to wear panties again. When she worked at the truck stops she would be in and out of so many trucks servicing the truck drivers that she did not bother to wear panties. She would normally be dressed in a skimpy top, short skirt and high heels. This way she wouldn't even have to get undressed. Just had to pull down her top to reveal her large breasts, then lift up her skirt and spread those legs.

There was an interesting case in Rockaway, NJ. When a 29 year old worker at Dunkin Donuts was arrested for prostitution during her 9pm to 5am shift. The code word to the cashier was "I would like an extra sugar". They would then drive around the corner park their car and wait for her. She would then take a 10-15 minute break to service the customer in the car. She was an average looking woman with brown hair, slightly overweight.

Las Vegas, Nevada has a slogan "what happens in Vegas stays in Vegas". Although prostitution is illegal, you will not have a problem finding a hooker. Most of them will advertise as escorts or dancers. They are advertised all over Las Vegas, from free magazines located in distribution bins to people on the streets handing out business cards or flyers. The street people would make clicking sounds with the cards to get your attention. They even have trucks with large mobile bill boards adverting women that will come direct to your hotel rooms. Vegas girls can cost you quite a bit though and you have to be careful of the agencies. They tell you that their rate is only $150 for the hour. When the girl arrives she takes the $150, and then tells you that the $150 is the agency fee and that any services are extra. That is why you will see some women will state in their ads that they are not an agency. The average price for a woman coming to your room in Vegas could cost you anything from $200 to $400. You can pick up a hooker who operates from the hotel bars for about $150. Others from websites like "back pages", advertise for as low as $100 for half an hour.

Don't be fooled by some of the low prices. As they say, you get what you pay for. I had a card from one of the street distributors that advertised a massage for only $40. I called the woman who gave me her description, mainly her height and color of her hair. I waited for about 45 minutes in anticipation in my hotel room at the Imperial Palace, wondering what this woman would look like. She sounded quite sexy over the phone. I had the choice of her, a brunette or her friend, a blond. Finally I heard the knock on the door. Excitedly I jumped up and ran over to the door to look through the peep hole. All I could see was darkness. I hesitated and soon heard the knock again. My curiosity got the better of me, so I unlocked the door to see what the bargain woman would look like. To my horror, there before me stood this 300 pound obese woman with the brunette hair and correct height as she had stated. For obvious reasons she had failed to tell me about her body. Before I could say anything she pushed her way into the room. At that point I had realized that she had blocked the peep hole on purpose. Although she was not my type, so to speak, she was a pleasant person. She was in her late forties, and a semi-retired hooker who had long past her prime working days. There was no way I was going to fuck her, so I settled for a good blowjob for the $40 plus a $20 tip.

In a Vegas bust a beautiful black woman with green eyes from Las Angeles was arrested in for prostitution while applying her trade in one of the hotels. She was a high class call girl who made as much as $7,000 a weekend in Vegas. She stated that if she did not make more than $1,500 a night she was not happy. Another plumpish white woman with shoulder length hair claimed she was in the business as she enjoyed sex, charging a client anything from $130 to $500.

If you want to go to where prostitution is fully legalized in Nevada, you have to head out to the rural counties towards Reno. There you will find fully operational whorehouses or as they also call them "cathouses". The prices can run you from $200 for 15 minutes all the way up to $10,000. Some of the famous Ranches include the Mustang, Cherry Patch, Pussycat, Chicken, Sheri's and Wild Horse Adult resort and Spa.

With the recent worldwide recession hard times has fallen to many Las Vegas residents, even affecting the supposed recession proof business of prostitution. In November 2010 a beautiful call-girl named Sandy told me that business had slowed down drastically, forcing her to give up her luxury three bedroom condo just off the strip, and settle for a small one bedroom condo instead.

A few years ago a couple was arrested for operating a high class prostitution business in Los Angeles. The women who worked for the organization were surprisingly from good families or who had professional jobs, which included single women, soccer moms, wives etc . . . These high end clients, mostly top business men, are referred to as "Hobbyists" while the women who provide the sexual services are referred to as "Providers". Most of the hobbyists are powerful or wealthy business men who want to take a break from the pressures of work or home. They just want a more personal time with the woman, to be treated well and for the woman to take control. These high class women can make as much as $12,000 in one day. A Provider who was a married woman cost a Hobbyist $25,000 which included an airfare for 12 hours, of which only 2 hours evolved sex. I am sure the husbands did not complain when their wives returned with a good days earning. Maybe a boost to their self esteem knowing how much another man is willing to pay to have sex with their wives.

During the Second World War in Pearl Harbor, the authorities and military welcomed women to work as prostitutes in the area to take care of all the soldiers who were stationed there or passing through. They encouraged these women to move there temporarily to supply a valued service to all the men in need.

In 2010 they were debating whether to decriminalize prostitution in Taiwan. One of the sticking points if decriminalized, was must a married woman get consent from her husband if she wants to become a prostitute? Some of the public claimed that this is discrimination. If a woman wanted to become a Minister she did not have to have consent from her husband. Another point made was if a woman needs consent from her husband to be a hooker, should the client also obtain consent from his wife to fuck one? With the decriminalization of prostitution, it would be classed as a "regular" job.

During the time that Nelson Mandela was imprisoned on Robin Island in South Africa, some of the white prison guards' wives would make extra money prostituting themselves to the single prison guards on the Island. Many of them had the consent from their husbands. This was an extra income the wives could make, as the prison guards did not make decent salaries. I can only imagine that the wives must have had a low going rate.

Fast forward to present day post apartheid. You will find many women in South Africa have opted for a career in prostitution. Even Nelson Mandela had tried to make prostitution legal. Many of them would advertise in the local newspapers with a going rate of about R300 ($43) and up. The classier women charge in excess of R500. During the 2010 World Cup Soccer there was an influx of prostitutes to South Africa, hoping to make a fortune. There are also whorehouses in some of the residential areas. They only mark them with a large sign with the house number. These houses normally house about 4-6 women a shift with a selection of White, Indian, Colored or African women. Some of the women in these houses are not the best of the best quality. The typical going rate is ($20) and up. With the Aids rate at about 20% of the population, one would have to be cautious. The rampant spread of Aids was a result of many African men refusing to wear condoms and the preference of dry sex. They would prefer the woman not to be lubricated naturally or unnaturally. Therefore during dry sexual contact lesions in the skin and transmission of the virus are more likely.

In Germany prostitution is totally legal, as the Germans are more liberal on sex matters than in most countries. It is estimated that the prostitution generates 30 billion Euros annually in Germany and there are about 400,000 sex workers in the country. There a brothel can only hire women with European passports. They have to pay 30 Euros per day for a sex worker license and another 30 Euros per day for management. Whatever they make is theirs. The average price is 60 Euros per half hour. Additional fees are for extras like anal, French kissing etc .... The brothels even cater for the disabled with wheel chair ramps and elevators. In Belgium it is said that more people visits brothels than the cinema.

Aug 2011 the Bonn city council in Germany decided to charge street prostitutes a parking meter tax. The idea was to make the street prostitutes pay taxes as the sexworkers do in a registered establishment like brothels. The workers can buy a ticket for the night from one of the vending style parking meters located on the street they wish to apply their trade. They would pay the equivalent of $8.70 for a night, the ticket would be valid for 8:15pm till 6am. Failure to purchase a ticket can result in a fine or been banned from practicing prostitution. They plan to collect an estimate amount of $270,000 annually from the street sexworkers. Street prostitution in Bonn is restricted to certain areas.

Many escorts or call girls used to advertise on Craigslist until they were forced to pull there "erotic" ads due to a CNN documentary that aired in 2010. The documentary was titled "Selling the girl next door", which mostly dealt with under age prostitutes. When Craigslist pulled their erotic ads, Backpage.com had an increase of one million dollars a month in "erotic" ads. They too were soon forced to pull their erotic ads. Just goes to show you how much money circulates in the sex business. It is believed that Holland with only a population of 16 million generates a gross revenue of 660 million Euro ($865 million) a year in the sex industry, which mostly comes from tourists.

After reviewing all the places around the world, Curacao must rank among the cheapest and best value for money. You tend to be spoilt by the low Campo price of $28 for half an hour. After paying these prices it is a major adjustment to get back to paying regular prices. Most first world countries a woman will cost you $100 to $150 for half an hour and $180 to $300 for a full hour.

CHAPTER 15
FANTASIES AND FETISHES

Many people have fantasies or fetishes, but only a few act on them. I once read in an advice column where a man had a certain fantasy he wanted to explore and the advice he received was: "Best keep it as a fantasy, don't act it out". My basic rule is that as long as it does not harm or offend anyone and that minors are not involved, go for it.

One of the most popular fantasies among men is to have a sex with two women. Some find it difficult to arrange. The problem with arranging this with working girls is that most of them would fake the sex with another woman. They would pretend to be eating her pussy, but in fact is only pushing her mouth onto the pussy, no tongue in play. Having said that, you can find the odd hooker who is really into this and will actually eat and suck that pussy. The best is to ask them before making the deal, if they will actually be fucking and sucking for real. I personally have experienced this many, many times both paying for it and having it for free.

Another that men enjoy, not a personal favorite of mine, is anal sex. Also know as Greek. Most women that do allow this do expect some extra cash for this service. There are some that do it for their own enjoyment.

I was with a tall olive skinned Colombian woman at Campo one day. I was lying down on the bed as she mounted me. While telling me to relax and enjoy I felt her pussy very tight but not well lubricated. She slid slowly up and down my cock, with her enjoying every stroke. I looked down towards her pussy only to find a vacant pussy hole and my cock well embedded in her tight ass. She either thought that I was into this or that she just loved getting fucked in the ass.

At Campo as you pass by the rooms, you will see all different types and sizes of dildos displayed on the window sills. These are used either for the woman to play with herself, while the man watches or some men opt to have the dildos used on them.

I suppose every man has their own fantasies or fetishes. Here are some of the stranger ones I have heard of:

A street hooker had a man who wanted her to go with him to the zoo and act like a monkey, making monkey sounds and then have sex with him. She turned him down.

One hooker did go through with this man's fantasy. He wanted to be wrapped in Saran™ wrap with only the head of his cock showing. He was then suspended upside down and had a dog lick his cock.

Most Latina women are not into heavy bondage or SM. Light bondage is something they would go for as some do stock handcuffs.

One year when visiting Campo it was Halloween. Many of the girls dressed up in costumes. This was a great night for fantasies. I don't know how or where the girls got the costumes from, but what a good site. There were nurses, school girls, policewoman, angels and fairies etc . . . Did not find my Hiawatha but did fuck a fairy that night. I was able to fuck her without damaging her wings. The fairy costume must have been a popular fantasy with the men, as she was able to fuck 10 men that night all before 12am.

I had a student respond to an ad I had placed in the local Internet classifieds. I was interested in trying out a Dutch woman in exchange for cash. A local black student responded as she was curious to experience being paid for sex. She was a slightly plumpish woman about 19 years old. Not what exactly what I was looking for, but decided to go along for the experience. We settled on a $40 price. What surprised me was her fantasy. She said she always fantasized about being a slave girl, getting fucked by her master. She was on all fours on the bed with me ramming her doggie style. She was blaring out "fuck me master, fuck me". I was a bit uneasy going along with this one with all the racial tension of the past. Have to say she enjoyed it.

There are plenty more fetishes to cover. Here are some abbreviations and terms that a Dominatrix or Hookers use for services they provide:

69 (mutual oral)
Anal (Anal sex)
A-Level (5 star escort)
BJ (Blowjob)
BBBJ (Bareback Blowjob)
CBJ (Covered Blow Job; Oral sex with a condom)
CD (Cross Dressing)
CID (Come In Deep)
CIF (Come In Face)
COB (Come On Body)
COF (Come On Face)
Completion (Oral to completion)
Covered (Covered blowjob)
DATY (Dinner At The Y)
DFK (Deep French Kissing)
DSL (Dick Sucking Lips)
DT (Dining at the Toes English Spanking)
Doggie (Sex style from behind)
Duo (Sex with two hookers; Threesome with the client)
Extraball (Have sex many times)

FK (French kissing, Kissing with tongue)
GFE (Girl Friend Experience)
HJ (Hand Job)
Incall (You meet the girl at their place)
LT (Long Time; Usually overnight)
LTR (Long Term Relationship)
O-Level (Oral sex)
Outcall (Hooker visits you)
OWO (Oral without a condom)
Rimming (licking anus)

Besides the threesome being two women and one man, there are some who prefer the threesome to be two men and one female (a favorite preferred by some women). This threesome can involve the woman receiving vaginal sex and anal sex at the same time. Juan Carlos told me a story when he had one of these occasions with a friend of his. His friend had taken the back door and him from the front, when his friend remarked "hey I can feel your dick inside her". The other way is to have the woman give one a blow job while the other man fucks her. This can be done in doggie style, missionary or any preferred position where she can receive the second cock in her mouth. Some men would go as far as placing both their cocks in the pussy at the same time, but only if her pussy can stretch that wide. Have even heard about the woman's armpits been used.

As I mentioned before that many of the women at Campo nowadays display all different types and sizes of dildos in their windows. I don't know if there is a higher demand for this fantasy or if more women are getting into the act. Some men like to receive instead of giving. Whether this is experimental or a kinky desire they enjoy. The woman wears a strap on dildo and screws the guy up the ass or penetrates him with dildos while stroking his cock. A working woman did mention to me that they do put condoms on the dildos for hygienic reasons and to help with lubrication.

It is a known fact that a man does have a g-spot up his ass. This is the prostate gland, that when rubbed can cause a man to ejaculate. A man can even ejaculate during a routine prostate exam. Many hookers or masseuses do offer prostate massages. They typically place a condom on their finger, then insert up the anus and massage the prostate area. This is located not far from the entrance towards the front. They would play with his cock while they are massaging. This is a very popular demand in the Far East, but I am sure enjoyed by many men all over the world. Not to worry, this is not a gay thing if you want to try it.

Panties have always intrigued or turned men on, especially if they have been worn. Even the sight of panties seen up a skirt or a protruding g-string at her back, is a turn on for most men. Some men request to wear the woman's panties themselves while they fuck the woman or have them jerk them off. Cumming on panties can also be a fantasy that some women will allow for a few extra bucks. Fucking a woman with her panties still on, pulled to the side exposing her pussy opening, allowing the man to insert his cock is also desirable. Some woman will advertise the selling of used panties on the Internet. In the days before the internet you would find these ads in men's nude magazines. I saw an ad on a Toronto website where the woman would claim she will place the panties up her pussy and leave it there for 24 hours, before shipping them off to you.

The site of seeing a woman's panty is a treat for almost all men. Soon after 911 I was waiting in the security line at Miami airport. The line stretched all the way from terminal D to C. As I was standing in line I noticed a young woman sitting on the floor rearranging her suitcase. Out the back of her jeans her g-string was clearly exposed. The line was moving very slowly so I had a great view point for my observation. I watched many men react as they walked past. The woman totally unaware of the attention she had created. Married men or those with their girlfriends would quickly sneak a look, while some men on their own would just stop and stare. It was quite amusing to watch this and helped pass the time while in line. Once again Miami international airport welcomed me with a panty flash. As I was waiting for my baggage at the conveyer belts I noticed a beautiful well tanned woman (probably Cuban American) on the opposite side. She had sexy smooth legs, and was wearing high heeled wedge shoes. Well to my delight she decided to squat down, probably to rest. With knees apart she gave me a clear view of her pink panties. I looked around to see other men enjoying the "Welcome to Miami" view.

A pair of panties did get me into trouble years ago. A few of my friends and I at Campo decided to play a little game. We randomly selected a room number for each other. We would then go to the room that was chosen and have sex with the hooker no matter what she looked like. We had to return with her panties as proof that you were with her. Later that night I arrived back home. My wife was asleep. I realized I still had the pair of panties in my pocket so I quickly hid it in a place I knew she should not look. I placed them in my winter jacket pocket, knowing that I would not use the jacket anytime in the Caribbean.

Months had past when my wife and I were visiting Amsterdam during winter on the way to South Africa. The panty story was long since forgotten by now. My wife was wearing my winter jacket at the time and placed her hands in the pocket. To my utmost surprise she pulled out her hand holding the panties and curiously asked me "what is this?". I was totally caught off guard. After rattling my brain for a few seconds, I decided to tell her the truth that it was a game my friends and I had played. The truth was that I did not fuck the woman that night that stood in the doorway of the number I was given. She was not desirable or to my taste. So I offered her about $10 to buy one of her panties, which she obliged. It took a while before I could convince my wife it was just a game and that no sex had conspired. Luckily we were in the sexual capital of the world, so we were soon distracted and the panty discovery soon forgotten.

Chapter 16
What Makes a Good Hooker

By no means am I trying to encourage women to become prostitutes. If a woman decides to go into the business of her own free will and asked me for advice, this is what I I'd say or tell her.

If a woman decides to become a hooker, there are quite a few points she should consider that can help her become a successful hooker. Many successful hookers have taken the business approach to ply their trade. A woman I knew who decided to get in the business in her forties had a Bachelor degree in business. She knew her education would finally pay off and help in her new venture. She approached it in a well organized business manner. Her only worry was that her pussy would stretch from all the large thick cocks she would have to fuck.

As Donald Trump would say "If you do something you enjoy, you will be successful at it". So if you love sex this is definitely a good career choice. I mentioned earlier in the book about Adriana. She got into the business purely because she loved and enjoyed sex. She would not focus on the money, instead get so deeply evolved in the sexual desires of her clients. The money then naturally came in because of satisfied customers. Most of her clients would pay her much more than the going rate with the great service she gave, and that she did it with so much passion.

The first thing a woman needs to remember is that her body is her main business asset. Keeping fit and in shape can help keep her body attractive to her customers. Don't over exert yourself. Take small vacation breaks when possible. Eat healthy and exercise. There is nothing worse than having a sexy woman in the room dressed in a tight dress, but as soon as the dress comes off, a fat belly rolls out. I had one of these women, she looked so sexy when dressed, but as soon as the dress was removed, the moment was dampened. Out flopped a belly and love handles. Please women work on that stomach.

I am not saying the overweight women can't make money. You don't have to look like a movie star, just find out how to maximize your looks to convey sex appeal. There have been many TV shows that have performed makeovers for women without having any surgery. It can be just a matter of wearing the right clothes and having the right makeup done. To be fair, different men have different tastes in women as well.

A woman once asked me what she should wear when she ventured out to become a high class hooker in a hotel. I told her not to dress too slutty or tarty. Be sophisticated but sexy. Typical sexy office attire can work well in this case. You don't want to stand out as a hooker, but sexy enough to attract a man's attention.

Wearing an ankle chain can be very sexy. Ankle chains also referred to as anklets in the past, were used by whores to signal that that were available for business. In ancient Baal times the ankle chain was worn as way to identify who the prostitutes were during the satanic worship. Nowadays this is not the case. They are worn by women of all walks of life. I think an ankle chain worn is very sexy, classy and a turn on for most men. Some men have commented to me that a choker necklace worn by a woman is a turn on for them. Juan Carlos had commented to me after seeing a porn movie where a boss had given his secretary a choker necklace to symbolize that she was now his sexual slave, he would be turned on by any woman that wore a choker. Most people believe the choker was worn mostly by slaves, but it was fashionably worn in the old days by the French and English high society, along with Queens, Princesses and other Royals. Many cultures around the world throughout history have worn chokers. The next and probably one of the most important points is "SERVICE". If you plan to have repeat business, it is very important to give good service and have a pleasant attitude towards your customers. There is nothing worse than having a woman who rushes you. As I stated before we classed these women as "she is just business". I have found many of the younger women new in the business mistakenly start out like this. It might be that they think their young tight bodies are all that the customer wants. With more experience they soon learn if they want a longer career in the sex business . . . . service counts.

Good hygiene is of utter most importance. A foul odor will definitely not bring repeat business, unless this is a man's fetish. King Louis the XVI who was guillotined during the French revolution was one such man. Apparently he would like his women not to bath for days or even weeks before he would have sex with them. I have noticed that most Latin American women practice good hygiene. They use a feminine hygiene liquid soap called "Lemisol" to wash themselves. After sex they would sit on the toilet, spread their legs. Using a plastic cup they would fill it with water from the wash basin beside them. Soak their pussy with water, apply the Lemisol and gently massage their gold mine. After rinsing and drying, their pussy is fresh and clean for the next client. Sometimes they will use this soap to wash your dick. It leaves a refreshing tingling feeling on your balls and cock. A sort of menthol feeling. It would be great to even get your girlfriend or wife to use this soap. In Dominican Republic they even use it as a shower gel. I have tried this. Your whole body feels cool and fresh.

Just as if you are going on a date, a hooker needs to practice good oral hygiene. At Campo most girls brush their teeth after each client. Bad breath can scare away a potential customer. Even a quick rinse with mouth wash is fine.

Never rush into the sex act. Talking or making your customer feel relaxed and comfortable is always a good thing. Undressing the customer can be a simple sexy gesture that most men like. The man loves to be treated like a King. Eye contact is good. Show the customer you are interested in him and pay attention to his requests. Some might just be verbal fantasy talk that gets him horny. Play along with him even though he might not want to actually act it out. You will find that you be playing the role of many professions or characters. Girlfriend, wife, marriage/relationship councilor, shrink, sex therapist, friend, dominatrix, submissive, slave, actress, mistress, lover, teacher, student and many more.

There are many forms of prostitution: Call girls, escorts, street hooker, brothel hookers, bar hookers, truck stop hookers, windows (Amsterdam), hotel lobby hooker, and independent hookers. The independent hookers offer either in call (the client goes to their place), or outcall (the girl goes to the clients' house or hotel room). The independent or escorts mostly advertise in classified ads in newspapers or on the

Internet. Some women don't like to be classed as hookers, prostitute or escort, but instead opt to be a mistress having just one client or only a few.

One of the safer ways to start would be with an escort agency, as some of them screen their clients. Most times you are accompanied to the location by a driver. The agency then recommends you call in upon arrival and departure. A legal brothel can also be a safe place to work as they would have security and even panic buttons in the rooms. Campo rooms are equipped with such panic buttons.

If I was a female hooker, I would opt for high class call girl. You will be amazed at how much some men are willing to pay for sex or for just the company. The rates can reach into the thousands of dollars. A female magazine writer who was writing an article on one of Nevada's brothel decided to pack up her day job and become one of the hookers. She called up her boss and told him she was quitting, but did promise to finish the article. Within her first week she had a daytime client who paid $3,000 to be with her.

Men are hunters, they will always chase after something they can't have. It is a personal accomplishment to conquer the woman, no matter how much it costs him. Being a high class call girl you have to learn to set your price so that you don't scare off potential clients with too high of a price or come off too cheap.

They always say any woman has her price. I put this to test with an innocent 18 year old virgin. Testing her slowly increasing the offer to see when her breaking point would be. When I reach $1,000 she started contemplating it. I did not go through with the sexual transaction as I personally knew this woman. Sometime later I eventually was able to get my way without paying her. Not a full sexual encounter. I had her dance and partly strip for me. She wore a blindfold so she could not see me jerk off while she lifted up her skirt flashing her panties. She sensually danced to the Latino music in front of me until I shot my load all over my chest.

As any business it will take time to build up a good clientele. A Canadian woman who mostly did outcalls to hotels explained this to me. She would operate between two cities. It took her about three months to build up a good client base between the two cities. The reason behind working with two cities was that most clients would need a change after a while. So when she thought that the regulars were at the point when they need a change, she would move back to the other city. By that time that city clients will be anxious to have her back.

If a woman with no experience wanted to become an independent call girl, I would recommend starting at an escort agency to learn ins and outs about the business. An experienced hooker once told me that over time she learnt how to screen her customer over the phone by asking certain questions and analyzing their answers. Unfortunately I did not get the chance to hear what kind of questions she would ask. Her resume showed that she went from been a medical worker to a stripper and ending up as a hooker over the years, mostly a result of her drug usage.

Try stay away from draws of drugs. If you need to take drugs to help you perform the act of prostitution, then maybe this is not the work for you. You just have to take a look at the street crack whores to see how their lives have spiraled out of control. I see these women on the street corners and wonder what clientele they are attracting. Most legal brothels or high class escort agencies will state in their job opportunity ads, that substance abuse is not tolerated.

Treat your profession as a career and set financial goals. Remember that this is a profession you may be forced to retire at a younger age than the normal retirement age of 60. But I have seen a 60 year old woman still applying her trade. I have to say by 60 year olds pictured on the internet, she didn't look to bad and had some class.

As you progress in age the term used is "mature". You will find that most of the mature hookers cater more and more to fetishes and fantasies that some of the younger women are not willing to perform or have no experience in.

A Massage parlor can also be a safe place to work. They would normally call it a massage with a "happy ending". The rooms are low light, soft sensual music playing in the background. The massage starts with the client lying on your stomach. This is normally how an erotic massage starts. In the Caribbean or South America if a masseuse makes you lie down first on your back, that is an indication that it is just a professional massage not an erotic one. Please note that in other parts of the world a professional massage, can start with the customer lying on his stomach. They normally ask the client if he wants the massage with oil. After massaging your back and legs for a while, once the client turns over the woman normally goes straight to the erotic massage or the "happy ending" begins. They would apply oil to the man's cock and balls, then proceed to skillfully rub the balls and cock until the man explodes freely squirting his cum over the woman's hands, arm or all over his body. She will then wipe up all the cum, using a hot moist towel or the sanitizing wet wipes. Leaving the clients cock and balls cleanly fresh.

As I mentioned before some of the top earners in Campo have made over $20,000 in three months. In Canada a woman working in a massage parlor can make as much as $2,000 a week, provided they are willing to offer a full service. A "full service" means massage, female totally naked and sex included. This can cost you about $180. Of which the house takes the $40 room fee and the balance of $140 goes to the girl. I met a beautiful Russian woman who would get up to 5 customers a night requesting the full service. On a slow night she would normally only get 2 full services and a few hand jobs to do. She said she made a comfortable living doing a job she enjoyed.

I was told about a woman who made as much as $10,000 in one night. She was an independent call-girl who operated out of her home. That night the neighbors complained about all the cars that were pulling up all night. Her going rate was $500, so based on that she must have had at least 20 men.

High class escorts on the internet can offer their services from $300-$500 an hour, $1,000-$3000 for the whole night. I have to say these are normally beautiful model looking women.

Remember your body is the most important asset to your business, so look after it and in return it will look after you financially.

CHAPTER 17
EPILOGUE

Prostitution is one of the oldest professions, with records dating back to 2400 BC. The ancient Sumerian people had the word "kar-kid" for female prostitutes back then. There will always be women willing to exchange sex for money. The demand will always be there. There are men from all walks of life that at some time have been guilty of having paid money for some form or another for a bit of pussy.

There is even a form of prostitution in the animal kingdom. Nature observers in Africa have witnessed female chimpanzees submitting to sex with their male counterpart in exchange for food.

With the introduction of Viagra, Cialis or other generic sexual enhancing drugs these days, this must have caused an increase in men frequenting women for sexual services. There is a joke with the claim that both Viagra and Cialis state on their labels "Seek immediate medical help for an erections lasting more than 4 hours". It should read "seek a hooker".

Other stimulants like poppers, rush or amyl nitrate are known to make sex great and increase orgasms. Amyl nitrate is a prescription drug. But rush or poppers contain isobutyl nitrate which is available over the counter at most sex shops. As a friend told me sniff it just before you cum and you will empty out your balls. I did try it along with a dietary supplement called "Stiff Nights" which lasts up to 72 hours. After having great sex and several masturbations, I had to stop as I actually ran out of cum over a 24 hour period.

I had a telephone interview with a man who was working on a research project for a University and the Government on "Johns", men who have paid for sex. The last question dealt with my views on why I think prostitution should be legal from a moral and family stand point. One of the biggest problems or complaints about prostitution is the illegal activity surrounded with this business, notably connections to the drug business, underage girls and organized crime. I explained to him my philosophy based on a personal story. When grew up in South Africa it was during apartheid and its conservative ways. It was illegal to purchase or be in possession of magazines like Playboy or Hustler. There was a big demand for these scarce materials. If you managed to buy a used one the pages were normally crumpled up or sticking to each other.

When I moved to Curacao these magazines were readily available. In my 20 years living in Curaçao I can confidently say that I have only bought two or three of these magazines. So if prostitution is totally legal it will not entice those who indulge in illegal or risky activity for a rush. The other point is that when prostitution is fully legalized, it should be regulated and controlled. From experience around the world, those places that have legal regulated prostitution, experience less criminal activity that those places that where illegal prostitution thrives.

The question always arises, why men pay for sex. One of the most legitimate ones is that you pay for the sex without any strings attached. If you were to walk down the street with your wife or girlfriend and see the hooker you had just fucked the night before, it is an unwritten code of conduct that she will not greet or acknowledge you.

In the movie "Risky Business" starring Tom Cruise, he played a character named Joel. He sells the idea by stating "Do the simple math on how much it will cost you to wine and dine a girl with the hope that you will get laid. You can end up been out of pocket for quite a bit and still not get laid, this way you are guaranteed to get laid for less."

With most men I think it is that sense of danger or rawness of knowing you are fucking a woman that is there just for the sake of been fucked. Some men have the desire to only go for street hookers as it is a turn on for them to see a woman standing on that street corner, dressed in a mini and high heels prancing along just waiting to be fucked for money. Perhaps it is something primal happening within the man. Others go looking for something they cannot get at home.

If a woman had to ask me for advice on what she can do to stop her husband or boyfriend from going to see a prostitute. I would tell her to be inventive. Try a bit of role playing, be the slut in bed that your man desires. I believe an open dialogue between couples is always the best solution. Don't be afraid to ask or tell your partner what you like or don't like. Last but not least, gentlemen be fair to your female partner, try and be romantic at times. Cater to her needs, not just your own.

A woman I knew had a customer who told her he would tell his wife that he had been with a prostitute. At first the wife would be very angry with him, but would later calm down and ask for a detailed description on the encounter. After hearing about the encounter she would get turned on and they would end up having great makeup sex. There are women that know their husbands are seeing a hooker, but are ok with it as long as they are not made aware of this in public or kept a secret from her. They pretend it does not happen or are just okay with it. This is common with some Latin American women.

I've been fortunate to have many conversations with the working girls over the years and in some cases getting to know them in depth or on a personal level. I have to say I have the utmost respect for them. No matter how degrading or low opinion some people have of these working women, they are all human and some have a heart of gold.

Some women have told me that working as a hooker has boosted their self esteem. Notably they thought that they were not pretty enough or not on par with other beautiful women. The fact is there are men so willing to have sex with them, and they are prepared to pay good money to have sex with these women. Men often tell them that they are beautiful and seeing the customer get an erection for them is a definite boost, knowing well that either their look or just their presence has excited the man.

There are many women who have met their future husbands in while working in a brothel and have gone on to living normal family lives. If I met up with one of these women later in life, out of respect for them I have never mentioned or acknowledged to them or their husbands that I knew them from that past when, they engaged in the sex business. Of course I would also never mention if I had used their services before.

One of the most famous prostitutes ever to progress in life has to be Ella Peron. The First Lady of Argentina, the wife of then President Peron from 1946 'till her death in 1952. It is believed she started as a prostitute in her earlier years as a way to get out of poverty and help her progress as an actress. She was beloved by many in Argentina, Latin America and other parts of the world. She inspired the 1996 movie "Evita" starring Madonna and Antonio Banderas.

There are many men who fall in love with these women. A comment Juan Carlos had heard from Gavin "She must love me, she called me *Papi*". Gavin would sing love songs to this particular girl as he fucked her. One song he would sing to her was the song by Lionel Richie and also sung my Kenny Rogers "Lady".

"Lady, I'm your knight in shining armor and I love you.

You have made me what I am and I am yours.

My love, there's so many ways I want to say I love you

Let me hold you in my arms forever more . . . ."

Some hookers are known to be very jealous, especially after you have been with them a few times and they then see you going with another hooker. Some men would hide or sneak around so that their regular does not see them going for another woman. This is a bit ironic. On one side the men are afraid to be caught cheating on one hooker by another hooker, and on the flip side these women are in the business for money not love.

Some men will pay a woman at campo to keep their door and pussy closed for business. They would pay heavily for this and engage in an "Girlfriend Experience". Some of these girls do obey their "boyfriend", while others would sneak a fuck when they could.

Luz, a 24 year old Colombian, was the most down to earth genuine whore I have ever met. She was the woman who would thank you for fucking her so that she could make money to help support her family. She was a woman I felt very comfortable with and I am sure many men including myself would have no problem with her becoming their wife, knowing well what work she had done. This is a woman you know you can love and receive love back.

I did fall in love and had a serious relationship with one of these women. This was a real life story that resembles the movie "Pretty Woman" that starred Julia Roberts and Richard Gere. The woman was Lucia who is mentioned throughout the book. I was separated at the time in my mid thirties. I was very attracted to her beauty, tallness and fun character. Our relationship started while she was still working at Hotel Stellaris. When she had enough customers for the night or things were quiet, she would call me to pick her up, normally around 12am, so she could spend the rest of the night with me. I would normally drop her off on my way to work in the morning and sometimes pick her up after my work, making sure she was back at the hotel at 8pm to start her nightly work.

There was even a romantic time we stood together barefoot on the beach, our feet grounded to earth in the sand by Avila Hotel round 11pm. It was a clear moonlit night, a calm Caribbean Sea glistened with the small waves brushing up on the beach. I held her in my arms kissing and hugging each other. Her hair was flowing freely in the light wind. At that moment we promised each other that we will one day be together. After this stint in Curacao she said she wanted to stop prostitution and live a normal family life.

She did return back to Curacao and stayed with me for a while. Even attending a political fund raising party where we both were greeted by the Prime Minister of the Netherlands Antilles.

The big difference I did notice with having a girlfriend who was an ex hooker was that she was more acceptable to having sex at any time. I would wake up in the middle of the night horny, and she would gladly part those beautiful legs for me. I was still dealing with a rough separation and our relationship was put on hold. What saddened me was that one night I walked into the bar at Stellaris a few months later. I found her sitting at the bar. She had returned back to her old trade. When she saw me her beautiful eyes filled with tears. She was so ashamed that I had seen her return to prostitution after she had told me she wanted out. She later moved to Europe where we kept in contact for a while.

About twelve years later I decided to try locate her through the internet. Part of me hoping that we could still live up to the promise we had made on the beach that moonlit night back in Curacao. I was fortunate to locate her, but had reached her two months too late as she had just got married to an older gentleman. What was surprising to me is that just a few months ago she had spent her honeymoon only 15 minutes away from where I now live. So who knows what tomorrow will bring.

One night with friends I was sitting on the patio at Campo in 2010 with a bottle of White Label Scotch on the table, a bucket of ice and plastic cups. They would not serve you in glasses. Anyway, we were reminiscing about the good years of Campo. I remarked that there has been a generational change over my 21 year of knowing Campo. Most of the girls working now are probably daughters of the ones we had been with in the early nineties.

Slowly over the years you will see some of them returning back for the three month stints. After they reach their thirties they seem to disappear back into a life of which I am curious to know what has happened to them.

I have met some very interesting women over the years. Some I would safely say I would love to have them as my companion. I often think about Adriana the day we realized we were a perfect sexual match, when she said to me in Spanish "marry me, marry me papi". At the time I was seeping deeper and deeper in to sexual desires. Her comment shocked me back into reality at that very moment she told me to marry her. I have to say she is one of the ones that got away. I regret not keeping in touch with her as we had mutual sexual desires and fantasies. It was a time I had met my true sexual match. I had asked her what her ultimate sexual fantasy was. It turned out to be my ultimate fantasy. One we both never had the chance to experience. The fantasy and level of sexuality we both experienced is a subject worthy of a second book.

Last but not least, I you may wonder if the 22 year old Colombian woman Katy had managed to fulfill her fantasy of fucking a guy up the ass with a strap on. Well I returned to Campo hoping to catch her before her three months was up. I tried calling her on the number she gave me and even went to her room. I was told she had left. If I ever get the answer to this I will post it on my website at **myputas.com**. I suppose you would have thought I was going to tell you "yes she did act on her fantasy and I must say it was a very painful experience for me."

THE END

www.ingramcontent.com/pod-product-compliance
Lightning Source LLC
Chambersburg PA
CBHW061247280526
45784CB00002B/671